The Juice Lady's

REMEDIES

FOR THYROID DISORDERS

CHERIE CALBOM, MS, CN

SILOAM

Most CHARISMA HOUSE BOOK GROUP products are available at special quantity discounts for bulk purchase for sales promotions, premiums, fund-raising, and educational needs. For details, write Charisma House Book Group, 600 Rinehart Road, Lake Mary, Florida 32746, or telephone (407) 333-0600.

THE JUICE LADY'S REMEDIES FOR THYROID DISORDERS
by Cherie Calbom
Published by Siloam
Charisma Media/Charisma House Book Group
600 Rinehart Road
Lake Mary, Florida 32746
www.charismahouse.com

Cover design by Justin Evans

Visit the author's website at www.juiceladycherie.com.

Library of Congress Cataloguing-in-Publication Data:
An application to register this book for cataloging has been submitted to the Library of Congress.
International Standard Book Number: 978-1-62998-204-5
E-book ISBN: 978-1-62998-585-5

This book contains the opinions and ideas of its author. It is solely for informational and educational purposes and should not be regarded as a substitute for professional medical treatment. The nature of your body's health condition is complex and unique. Therefore you should consult a health professional before you begin any new exercise, nutrition, or supplementation program or if you have questions about your health. Neither the author nor the publisher shall be liable or responsible for any loss or damage allegedly arising from any information or suggestion in this book. Names and details of testimonials of some individuals mentioned in this book have been changed, and any similarity between the names and stories of individuals described in this book to individuals known to readers is purely coincidental.

The statements in this book about consumable products or food have not been evaluated by the Food and Drug Administration. The recipes in this book are to be followed exactly as written. Neither the publisher nor the author is responsible for your specific health or thyroid needs that may require medical supervision. The publisher and the author are not responsible for any adverse reactions to the consumption of food or products that have been suggested in this book.

Portions of this book were previously published by Siloam as *The Juice Lady's Living Foods Revolution*, ISBN 978-1-61638-363-3, copyright © 2011; *The Juice Lady's Weekend Weight-Loss Diet*, ISBN 978-1-61638-656-6, copyright © 2011; *The Juice Lady's Big Book of Juices and Green Smoothies*, ISBN 978-1-62136-030-8, copyright © 2013; and *The Juice Lady's Remedies for Asthma and Allergies*, ISBN 978-1-62136-601-0, copyright © 2014.

While the author has made every effort to provide accurate Internet addresses at the time of publication, neither the publisher nor the author assumes any responsibility for errors or for changes that occur after publication.

15 16 17 18 19 — 9 8 7 6 5 4 3 2 1

Printed in the United States of America

CONTENTS

INTRODUCTION ix

1 WILL I EVER BE WELL AGAIN? MY STORY 1
The Event That Took My Breath Away 2

2 THE LITTLE GLAND WITH BIG INFLUENCE 8
Thyroid Disorders 10
Do You Have a Suboptimal Thyroid Disorder? 10
Low Thyroid Health Quiz 11
Toxins 14
Food Allergies and Thyroid Function 16
Radiation 17
Other substances 19
Many Thyroid Conditions Are Due to Adrenal Gland
Problems 19
What Causes Adrenal Fatigue? 20
Adrenal Fatigue Followed My Attack 21
Lifestyle Factors That May Contribute to Adrenal Fatigue 23

3 GETTING BACK TO BETTER THAN
NORMAL 24
Almost Miraculous 25
Live to Your Full Potential 27
How to Achieve a Good Weight With
Hypothyroidism 29

4 WHAT YOU DON'T KNOW MAY BE
   KILLING YOUR THYROID 31
      Psychological factors. 31
      Dietary factors 32
         Are Nonstick Pans Affecting Your Thyroid?. 32
      What to Avoid. 34
      Sugar of all types 34
      Goitrogens. 34
      Polyunsaturated oils 36
      Food allergens. 37
      Gluten and casein. 37
      Some carbohydrates 38
      Iodized salt 39
      Halogens: chlorine, fluoride, and bromine. 39
      Mercury. 40
         Low Thyroid Linked to High Cholesterol. 41

5 NOURISH YOUR THYROID WITH LIVING
   FOODS 43
      Living Foods Every Day of Your Life 43
      Living Foods for Thyroid Health. 45
      Food Solutions for Those With Hypothyroidism 46
         Thermogenic Foods Rev Up Your Metabolism 48
      More Food Choices to Help Your Body Heal 49
         The Dirty Dozen List 49
         The Cleanest Foods List. 50

Simple Living Foods Meal Plan for Stressed
Adrenals and Thyroid 50
Sample diet plan (Day 1) 51

6 NUTRIENTS THAT SUPPORT THE
   THYROID............................... 53
Supplements That Help You Fight Thyroid
Disorders................................... 54
   Iodine.. 54
   Selenium... 54
   Zinc... 54
   Vitamin D.. 55
   Multivitamin 55
   Tyrosine... 55
   Glutathione.. 55
   Bladderwrack 55
Other Nutrients and What Foods to Juice Daily
to Benefit From Them 56
Herbs That Promote Healthy Thyroid Function 57

7 REV UP YOUR METABOLISM WITH
   FRESH JUICES AND SMOOTHIES 59
Not All Green Juices Are Good for Thyroid
Disorders................................... 60
All About Juicing 62
The Why and How of Juicing 67
   Guidelines for Juicing 68

8   JUICE, SMOOTHIE, AND LIVING FOODS
RECIPES TO HEAL YOUR THYROID 71

Juices 71

Smoothies 87

Living Foods Recipes 97

Breakfast 97

Salads 99

Main Courses 102

Healthy Desserts 108

NOTES 110

FOR MORE INFORMATION .114

The Juice Lady's health and wellness juice
retreats 114

INTRODUCTION

I BECAME KNOWN AS "the Juice Lady" on TV and in print because of a serendipitous request from the owners of the Juiceman company. I was living in Seattle, completing graduate school at Bastyr University (a school of natural medicine), when another graduate student and I were asked to write a little booklet containing juice recipes and nutrition information to accompany the Juiceman juicer. One thing led to another, and before long I was traveling around the country almost weekly as the Juice Lady, teaching people how to create nutritious juices that are guaranteed to renew health and vitality.

Since even before I decided to pursue my master's degree in nutrition science, I had a passionate personal interest in the benefits of high-quality nutrition. This is because it was juicing, detoxing, and eating whole organic foods that had brought me back to full health not only once, but twice. (Read my story in chapter 1.) Now I want nothing more than to bring other people along with me on the journey to full life.

In this book I want to introduce you to the special benefits of juicing to improve or restore your thyroid function. People need this information. Too many of you are suffering from symptoms of thyroid disorders, and you don't know what's wrong. Doctors don't seem to be able to help you, and when they try, their prescriptions come with unwelcome side effects and symptoms of their own, not to mention high price tags.

Are you ready for something better? It's time for you to learn to make highly nutritious juices in your own kitchen. Juices and smoothies made from fresh vegetables, fruits, and other foods can help you regain your health and vitality—and keep you healthy for the rest of your life. Given the insidiousness of serious thyroid disease, easy alternatives to expensive and often futile medical interventions deserve your careful consideration.

Why go to the trouble of making your own juice? Why not just buy it? After all, stores are now stocked with a growing array of juices and other beverages made from organic, natural ingredients.

The primary reason is that you simply cannot get complete nutritional benefits from juice that is not freshly made, regardless of how carefully it was bottled and stored. Too many of the vitamins and other nutrients are lost or altered in juice that is not fresh, even when it has been produced from the finest ingredients. Most of the bottled fresh juice is pasteurized, meaning high heat is used, which kills vitamins, enzymes, and biophotons.

Another obvious reason is that your choices will be limited to whatever sells best. Only juice recipes that are commercially viable will be manufactured and sold at your local store. If you learn to make your own juices, smoothies, and other beverages, you will be able to pick and choose based not only on your personal health needs, but also on your taste preferences. You may never buy juice again once your taste buds sample their first sip of one of the juices in this book. Take a quick look at the last chapter, where you will find recipes using ingredients more varied and numerous than you will ever be able to try. After a while you will be creating your own special combinations of yummy, fresh ingredients.

Your digestive system will be able to absorb the nutrition quickly so that it can enter your bloodstream and begin to achieve its complex healing work. The vitamins, minerals, enzymes, phytochemicals, and more—all extracted from nature's own containers—will make you feel healthier almost instantly.

To focus on the nutritional needs of your thyroid, I have specially selected from my always-growing collection of recipes. There is a reason for every one of my choices and combinations, and I have tried to balance tastes and other personal preferences with the changing health needs of people like you, who don't have all day to work in the garden or stand at the kitchen counter, but who want to zero in on top-notch nutrition that is both healthful and healing.

Juice is both a noun and a verb. Anybody can learn to juice. To get started, all you need is a good juicer. (On my website, www.juiceladycherie.com, you will find recommendations for juicers.) Skim the recipes in this book until one of them catches your eye. Stock your refrigerator and pantry shelves and plug in your juicer. Within minutes you will take your first sip. Later in the day find another recipe and give it a try. After a couple of weeks of your new routine, I know you will be feeling better. Your sluggishness will disappear, and you will be able to make other important lifestyle changes. Before long you may be able to say no to synthetic thyroid hormones, and your troubling (even debilitating) symptoms will be a thing of the past.

Here's to your health! (With a big smile, I am raising a tall glass of the fresh juice. It's true—I never get tired of it!)

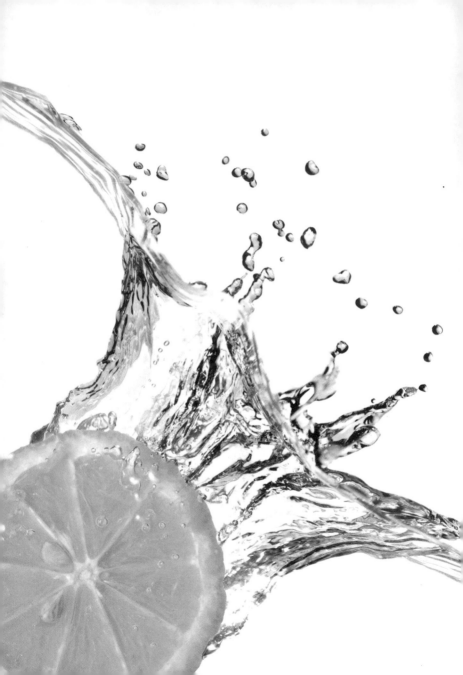

WILL I EVER BE WELL AGAIN? MY STORY

Sitting by the window one day in my father's home staring at the snow-topped mountains in the distance, I imagined that people were enjoying the hiking trails and perhaps someone was climbing the mountain that day. It was early June, and the weather was beautiful. I wished I had the strength to just walk around the block. But I was too sick and tired—I could barely walk around the house.

I had been sick for a couple of years and just kept getting worse. "Will I ever be well again?" I wondered. When I turned thirty, I had to quit my job. I had chronic fatigue syndrome and fibromyalgia that made me so sick I couldn't work. I felt as though I had a never-ending flu. Constantly feverish with swollen glands and perennially lethargic, I was also in constant pain. My body ached as though I'd been bounced around in a washing machine.

I had moved back to my father's home in Colorado to try and recover. But not one doctor had an answer as to what I should do to facilitate healing. So I went to some health food stores and browsed around, talked with employees, and read a few books. I decided that everything I'd been doing—such as eating fast food, granola for dinner, and not eating vegetables—was tearing down my health rather than healing my body. I read about juicing and whole foods, and it made sense. So I bought a juicer and designed a program I could follow.

I juiced and ate a nearly perfect diet of live and whole foods for three months. There were ups and downs throughout. I had days where I felt encouraged that I was making some progress but other days when I felt worse. Those were discouraging and made me wonder if health was the elusive dream. No one told me about detox reactions, which was what I was experiencing. I was obviously very toxic, and my body was cleansing away all that stuff that had made me sick. This caused some not-so-good days amid the promising ones.

But one morning I woke up early—early for me, which was around 8:00 a.m.—without an alarm sounding off. I felt like someone had given me a new body in the night. I had so much energy I actually wanted to go jogging. What had happened? This new sensation of health had just appeared with the morning sun. But actually my body had been healing all along; it just had not manifested until that day.

What a wonderful sense of being alive! I looked and felt completely renewed. With my juicer in tow and a new lifestyle fully embraced, I returned to Southern California a couple weeks later to finish writing my first book. For nearly a year I enjoyed great health and more energy and stamina than I'd ever remembered.

Then, all of a sudden, I took a giant step back.

The Event That Took My Breath Away

July fourth was a beautiful day like so many others in Southern California. I celebrated the holiday with friends that evening at a backyard barbecue. We put on jackets to insulate against the cool evening air and watched fireworks light up the night sky. I returned just before midnight to the house I was sitting for vacationing friends who lived in a lovely neighborhood not far from some family members. I was in bed just a bit after midnight.

I woke up shivering some time later. "Why is it so cold?" I wondered as I rolled over to see the clock; it was 3:00 a.m. That's when I noticed that the door was open to the backyard. "Wonder how that happened?" I thought, as I was about to get up to close and lock it. That's when I noticed him crouched in the shadows of the corner of the room—a shirtless young guy in shorts. I blinked twice, trying to deny what I was seeing. Instead of running, he leaped off the floor and ran toward me. He pulled a pipe from his shorts and began attacking me, beating me repeatedly over the head and yelling, "Now you are dead!" We fought, or I should say I tried to defend myself and grab the pipe. It finally flew out of his hands. That's when he choked me to unconsciousness. I felt life leaving my body.

In those last few seconds I knew I was dying. "This is it, the end of my life," I thought. I felt sad for the people who loved me and how they would feel about this tragic event. Then I felt my spirit leave in a sensation of popping out of my body and floating upward. Suddenly everything was peaceful and still. I sensed I was traveling, at what seemed like the speed of light, through black space. I saw what looked like lights twinkling in the distance. But all of a sudden I was back in my body, outside the house, clinging to a fence at the end of the dog run. I don't know how I got there. I screamed for help with all the breath I had. It was my third scream that took all my strength. I felt it would be my last. Each time I screamed, I passed out and landed on the cement. I then had to pull myself up again. But this time a neighbor heard me and sent her husband to help. Within a short time I was on my way to the hospital.

Lying on a cold gurney at 4:30 a.m., chilled to the bone, in and out of consciousness, I tried to assess my injuries, which was virtually impossible. When I finally looked at my right hand, I almost passed out again. My ring finger was barely hanging on by a small piece of skin. My hand was split open, and I could see deep inside. The next thing I knew, I was being wheeled off to surgery. Later I learned that I had suffered serious injuries to my head, neck, back, and right hand, with multiple head wounds and part of my scalp torn from my head. I also incurred numerous cracked teeth that resulted in several root canals and crowns months later.

I was so tired I could barely navigate through a day. My adrenal and thyroid glands were exhausted. The thyroid and adrenals are closely tied together. Often when the adrenal glands become exhausted, the thyroid gland is also affected. Adrenal fatigue usually develops over a period of time due to lifestyle, but it can also develop from acute stress, as in my case.

My right hand sustained the most severe injuries, with two knuckles crushed to mere bone fragments that had to be held together by three metal pins. Six months after the attack I still couldn't use it. The cast I wore—with bands holding up the ring finger, the one that had almost been torn from my hand, and various odd-shaped molded parts—looked like something from a science-fiction movie. I felt and looked worse than hopeless, with a shaved top of my head, totally red and swollen eyes, a gash on my face, a useless right hand, terrorizing fear, and barely enough energy to get dressed in the morning. I was an emotional wreck.

I couldn't sleep at night—not even a minute. It was torturous. Never mind that I was staying with a cousin and his family. There was no need to worry about safety from a practical point of view, but that made no difference emotionally. I'd lie in bed all night and stare at the ceiling or the bedroom door. I had five lights that I kept on all night. I'd try to read, but my eyes would sting. I could sleep for only a little while during the day.

But the worst part was the pain in my soul that nearly took my breath away. All the emotional pain of the attack joined up with the pain and trauma of my past for an emotional tsunami. My past had been riddled with loss, trauma, and anxiety. My brother had died when I was two. My mother had died of cancer when I was six. I couldn't remember much about her death—the memories seemed blocked. But my cousin said I fainted at her funeral. That told me the impact was huge.

I had lived for the next three years with my maternal grandparents and father. But Grandpa John, the love of my life, died when I was nine—the loss was immeasurable. Four years later my father was involved in a very tragic situation that would take far too long to discuss here, but to sum it up—it was horrific. He was no longer in my daily life. I felt terrified about my future. My grandmother was eighty-six. I had no idea how many more years she would live. The next year I moved to Oregon to live with an aunt and uncle until I graduated from high school.

As you can probably imagine, wrapped in my soul was a huge amount of anguish and pain with all sorts of triggers for emotional and binge eating. I know firsthand about eating-disorder behavior—binge eating and then not eating anything for a few days. I know what it is to get triggered emotionally and be clueless as to what set off an eating binge. Food is immediate comfort. It's often the first thing we turn to. It was for me. But not wanting to gain a lot of weight, I would then avoid food for a day or two after binge eating.

After the attack it took every ounce of my will, faith, and trust in God, deep spiritual work, alternative medical help, extra vitamins and minerals, vegetable juicing, emotional release, healing prayer, and numerous detox programs to heal physically, mentally, and emotionally. I met a nutritionally minded physician who had healed his own slow-mending broken bones with lots of vitamin-mineral IVs. He gave me similar IVs. Juicing, cleansing, nutritional supplements, a nearly perfect diet, prayer, and physical therapy helped my bones and other injuries heal.

After following this regimen for about nine months, what my hand surgeon said would be impossible became real—a fully restored, fully functional hand. He had told me I'd never use my right hand again and that it wasn't even possible to put in plastic knuckles because of its poor condition. But my knuckles did indeed re-form primarily through prayer, and function of my hand returned. A day came when he told me I was completely healed, and though he admitted he didn't believe in miracles, he said, "You're the closest thing I've seen to one."

The healing of my hand was indeed a miracle! I had a useful hand again, and my career in writing was not over as I thought it would be. My inner wounds were what seemed severest in the end and the hardest to heal. Nevertheless, they mended too. I experienced healing from the painful memories and trauma of the attack and the wounds from the past through prayer, laying on of hands, and deep emotional healing work. I called them the kitchen angels—the ladies who prayed for me around their kitchen table week after week until my soul was healed. I cried endless buckets of tears that had been pent up in my soul. It all needed release. Forgiveness and letting go came in stages and was an integral part of my total healing. I had to be honest about what I really felt and willing to face the pain and toxic emotions confined inside, and then let them go. Finally, one day after a long journey—I felt free. A time came when I could celebrate the Fourth of July without fear.

Today I know more peace and health than I ever thought would be possible. I have experienced what it is to feel whole—complete; not damaged, broken, wounded, or impaired; but truly healed and restored in body, soul, and spirit. And I'm not plagued with emotional eating anymore.

I have learned that my purpose was to love people to life through my writing and nutritional information to help them find their way to health and healing. If I could recover from all that had happened to me, they could too. No matter what anyone faced, there was hope. I want you to know that you are loved, and I send you my love between the lines of this book and with the juice and raw food recipes. There is hope for you.

You do not have to continue suffering the results of stress and exhaustion. No matter what challenges you face, there are answers that will heal your body, mind, and spirit. There's a purpose for your life, just as there was for mine. You need to be strong and well to complete your purpose. You can be greatly served by a positive mind and an optimistic attitude. With God's help and the latest nutritional data in this book, you can facilitate healing of your thyroid and experience abundant health. You can learn the right way to live your life to the fullest and finish well.

2

THE LITTLE GLAND WITH BIG INFLUENCE

THE THYROID IS a butterfly-shaped gland located at the base of your neck, just below your Adam's apple. It is one of the largest endocrine glands in your body, although it weighs less than an ounce, and the hormones it produces regulate the growth and rate of function of many other systems in your body. All aspects of your metabolism—from the rate at which your heart beats to how quickly you burn calories—are regulated by thyroid hormones.

It takes only a tiny change in hormone levels to cause big changes in your body. Hormonal imbalances cause the metabolism to slow down, leading to fatigue, weight gain, and a host of other problems. Laboratory tests can measure the hormone levels in your blood, urine, or saliva.

Thyroid problems are prevalent in this country, affecting as many as 20 percent of women and 10 percent of men. Many people go undiagnosed. But even for the people who learn that they have an overactive or underactive thyroid, it can be difficult to heal. Nevertheless, it's important to work on healing this gland because a healthy thyroid makes about 80 percent of the T4 hormone and 20 percent of the T3 hormone and traces of T2, T1, and calcitonin.

T4 is the major metabolism hormone and controls many

functions of the body. It's converted into T3 in the liver. T1 is thought to assist in the conversion process. If you produce too little T4, or if the T4 you produce is not being properly converted into T3, your whole system goes haywire—you suffer from a variety of symptoms such as low sex drive, fatigue in the morning, and weight gain. If you drastically cut calories to lose weight, calorie deprivation only serves to slow thyroid function further and causes more weight gain.

T3 is critical to your fitness because it sends messages to your DNA to rev up your metabolism and increase fat burning. It helps lower cholesterol, improves memory, keeps you trim, promotes growth or regrowth of hair, relieves muscle aches and constipation, and even helps with infertility in some people.

T2 is known to have a stimulatory effect on the enzyme that converts T4 to T3. It is effective in promoting liver metabolism and is involved in the activity of the heart muscle tissue. It also affects "brown fat"—the fat that is burned rather than stored in the body. Further, T2 can help in the breakdown of fat, making it an important hormone for weight loss and bodybuilding.

Calcitonin, a protein hormone, slows the release of calcium from the bones; it decreases bone breakdown and increases bone density. It also keeps blood levels of calcium low. There is a higher incidence of osteoporosis among people with hypothyroid, which would make sense since this gland regulates calcium metabolism. A 2007 study showed that calcitonin may protect postmenopausal women from osteoarthritis. In the study female rats were given salmon calcitonin; they showed less joint damage than those who were given a placebo.[1]

It's important to remember that using prescription thyroid hormone replacement is at times necessary, but it should only be used as a temporary solution while the actual cause of hypothyroid is explored. It's not advantageous to stay on thyroid medication indefinitely even though these hormones may reduce symptoms. It doesn't heal your thyroid gland. In fact, it has the opposite effect—your body will slowly produce less and less thyroid hormones because there are enough hormones in your system. Like your muscles, your thyroid will get weaker and weaker from lack of use. At the same time, you'll produce less calcitonin, and your bones will suffer.

Thyroid Disorders

When the thyroid gland does not produce enough thyroid hormone, symptoms can include extreme fatigue, depression, and weight gain. This is called hypothyroidism or underactive thyroid. Another form of thyroid disease causes the gland to produce too much thyroid hormone; this is known as hyperthyroidism or thyrotoxicosis. Symptoms of an overactive thyroid include irritability, nervousness, muscle weakness, unexplained weight loss, sleep disturbances, vision and eye problems. (A type of hyperthyroidism called Graves' disease affects about 1 percent of the population; it is a genetic autoimmune disorder.)

Do You Have a Suboptimal Thyroid Disorder?

A blood test may never indicate that you have a problem with this gland because these tests are designed to identify hypothyroid, not a suboptimal—just-a-bit-below-par—thyroid function. And yet nutritional remedies such as the juices and diets recommended in this book can be applied to the most benefit with low thyroid function.

Take the Low Thyroid Health Quiz, giving yourself a point for every symptom that describes you.

LOW THYROID HEALTH QUIZ

- Appetite problems—severely reduced or excessive
- Bipolarity (manic depression)
- Bloating or indigestion after eating
- Brittle nails
- Calcium deficiency
- Carpal tunnel syndrome
- Chronic mucus in head/nose (thyroid governs mucus production)
- Coarse, dry hair
- Cold hands and feet
- Constipation
- Decreased sweating
- Depression
- Difficulty concentrating
- Difficulty drawing deep breaths
- Dry mouth; drinking water doesn't help much
- Dry, rough skin
- Elevated cholesterol
- Emotionally unstable
- Enlargement of heart
- Fatigue/lack of energy
- Feeling of deep gloom for no apparent reason
- Fluttering in ears

- Forgetfulness
- Gasping for air occasionally
- Grinding teeth during sleep
- Grooves or ridges in nails
- Hair loss
- Heart pain
- Heart palpitations
- Hoarse throat
- Hypertension
- Impaired heart function
- Impotency
- Inability to "drag oneself from bed"
- Intolerance to closed, stuffy rooms
- Intolerance to cold or heat
- Irritability for no apparent reason
- Left arm weakness
- Lethargy
- Light menstrual flow
- Loss of hair on arms, underarms, legs, eyebrows, scalp
- Loss of hearing
- Loss of libido/low sex drive
- Loss of smell
- Low body temperature (below 97.6 degrees, resting)

- Miscarriages
- Mucus accumulation
- Muscle/joint problems—knees, elbows, etc.
- Need for fresh air
- Nervousness
- Numbness in fingers
- Occasional stinging in eyes
- Pain in diaphragm
- PMS
- Poor absorption of minerals
- Poor digestion of animal products
- Poor vision
- Premature deliveries
- Prolonged or heavy menstrual bleeding
- Puffy eyes
- Restlessness
- Sense of pressure (compression) on chest
- Shorter menstrual cycle
- Shortness of breath
- Shyness
- Sleep disturbances
- Slow-growing nails
- Slower heart rate
- Sluggish lymph drainage
- Spleen or liver problems

- Stiff neck
- Stillbirths
- Swelling—ankles, eyelids, face, feet, hands, lymph nodes, throat
- Tendency to cry easily
- Tenderness in lower ribs
- Thin, peeling nails
- Weight gain or difficulty losing weight
- White spots on nails (this can also be a zinc deficiency)

A score of twenty points or more may be indicative of low thyroid. Although the thyroid quiz can help you determine your thyroid health, ultimately the best method for diagnosis is clinical evaluation by a physician knowledgeable in thyroid health. I recommend you see a physician who can treat your condition holistically.

Toxins

The thyroid is a sentinel organ and is usually one of the first that is impacted by toxicity. According to the Functional Endocrinology Center of Colorado, chemicals such as phthalates, flame retardants, bisphenol A, dioxins, perfluorinated chemicals (PFOA), fluoride, mercury, perchlorate, thiocyanate, and pesticides can be very disruptive for thyroid function and seriously impact your health. Also, radiation can disrupt thyroid function. Let's take a closer look at several items on this list.

Phthalates increase the flexibility of plastics and are

commonly used in shower curtains, medical tubing, and plastic toys. They're also found in personal care items such as nail polish and lotion. Phthalates impact thyroid regulation by decreasing thyroid hormone receptor activity. Because of their widespread use and the fact that municipal water treatments don't remove them, they are showing up in drinking water.[2]

Polybrominated diphenyl ether (PBDE) is a flame-retardant chemical used in furniture foam, carpets, upholstery, clothing, toys, draperies, and electronics. This chemical readily accumulates in fat cells and has been linked to a decrease in TSH levels.[3]

Bisphenol A (BPA) is commonly used in polycarbonate water bottles, baby bottles, plastic toys, medical tubing, food packaging, and dental sealants. It has also been linked to disruption in thyroid receptors and thyroid function.[4]

Dioxins, including polychlorinated biphenyls (PCBs), polychlorinated dibenzodioxins (PCDDs), and polychlorinated dibenzofurans (PCDFs), are by-products from industrial processes such as chlorine paper bleaching, pesticide manufacturing, and smelting. Have you heard of Agent Orange used during the Vietnam War? Dioxins were part of this toxic biological weapon. Among other things, these chemicals interfere with production, transportation, and metabolism of thyroid hormones.[5]

Perfluorinated chemicals (PFOA [perfluorooctanoic acid] and PFOS [perfluorooctane sulfonate]) used in nonstick cookware, stain-resistant materials, and food packaging have been linked to decreased thyroid hormone levels.[6]

Perchlorate is a by-product of rocket fuel production that has shown up in drinking water, certain fruits and vegetables, and dairy products from cows that eat contaminated grass. It can inhibit iodine absorption, leading to low thyroid function.[7]

Thiocyanate is a chemical found in cigarettes and certain foods, and like perchlorate, it may inhibit iodine uptake and therefore lead to decreased production of the thyroid hormone.[8]

One of the best things you can do to avoid all this is to purchase only organic produce because pesticides sprayed on nonorganic foods often contain estrogenic compounds, which can affect the endocrine (hormonal) system that includes the thyroid. Avoid all plastic water bottles. Glass water bottles are best. Purchase a high-quality water purification system. Use an air filter in your home. Cook with only natural product cookware. Choose organic mattresses, bedding, towels, carpets, and fabrics for your home.

Clean with eco-friendly, natural products. And choose only fragrance-free, chemical-free, and organic personal care products. To make sure that you get rid of harmful toxins that have built up in your system, detox your body at least once, but preferably twice, a year.

FOOD ALLERGIES AND THYROID FUNCTION

When it comes to food-related allergies that impact the thyroid gland, it is not like eating a nut or a shrimp and getting an immediate reaction. The type of reaction that disrupts thyroid function is a delayed interaction with food antigens that can occur up to four days after eating the food.

The two most prevalent food-related reactions come from dairy and wheat. These two foods are known in alternative medicine to be highly correlated with autoimmune thyroiditis. Dairy and wheat gluten are often removed from diets of thyroid patients with good success. A study reported in

The Journal of Clinical Gastroenterology demonstrates that those allergic to gluten had a much greater risk of thyroid abnormalities.[9]

Radiation

It is known that radiation exposure increases the risk for thyroid cancer. Environmental exposure, such as that from nuclear power plants and radioactive fallout, and exposure from medical procedures are problematic. Airport scanners pose more of a problem for developing skin cancer. The risk of thyroid disease from radiation exposure increases in individuals who are iodine deficient. When you supplement your diet with iodine, it is taken up by the thyroid gland, which then blocks radiation uptake into the thyroid, reducing your risk for thyroid cancer—an epidemic in the United States likely due in part to excess CT scans combined with iodine deficiency. Potassium iodide is used to treat radiation emergency caused by exposure to radioactive iodides, but excess iodine can be harmful to health. However, water-soluble iodine seems to be much less problematic.

It's best to increase your iodine intake with food such as kelp powder, dulse, sea vegetables, seafood, and cranberries (all iodine rich) because radioactive iodine will drop into iodine receptor sites that have no iodine in them as a result of iodine deficiencies.

It's also important to increase your antioxidant intake. Radiation within the body generates massive amounts of damaging free radicals that can harm your DNA, which can lead to cancer a decade or two later. Therefore it's imperative to maximize your overall antioxidant intake by juicing and eating plenty of vegetables, especially the dark leafy greens, along with taking extra vitamins C and E, selenium, N-acetyl cysteine, alpha-lipoic acid, and coenzyme Q_{10}.

Unfortunately the antioxidant defense system of many Americans is in poor condition. Spirulina and chlorella are antioxidant rich and were used extensively by the Russians after the Chernobyl nuclear plant disaster. Miso is also protective and helpful to a person who has been exposed to radiation. It was used in Japan after World War II. Following the Nagasaki bombing, a group of macrobiotic doctors and their patients avoided radiation sickness and did not get leukemia by eating brown rice, miso, and seaweed.[10]

Juice more chlorophyll-rich foods such as wheatgrass, barley grass, kale, collard greens, beet greens, Swiss chard, parsley, rapini, kohlrabi leaves, and dandelion leaves, which help to strengthen cells, transport oxygen, and detoxify the blood and liver, helping to bind up polluting elements and stimulate RNA production. (I recommend juicing them because you can consume much more by juicing than just eating the plants.) Also, eat and juice more sulfur-containing vegetables, including broccoli, cabbage, mustard greens, and garlic, which combine with heavy metals and prevent free-radical damage. Cilantro helps to remove heavy metals and radioactive materials from the brain. Juice up a large handful of cilantro each day.

Take baths with baking soda and magnesium salts. Uranium will bond with sodium bicarbonate (baking soda). This will help to protect the kidneys and cleanse the body. To combat radioactive fallout or exposure to radiation, start by using one pound of baking soda in a bath; add to that magnesium in the form of bath flakes, Dead Sea salt, or Epsom salts.

Other substances

Caffeine and alcohol. It's important to avoid coffee, black tea, green tea, sodas, chocolate, and all alcoholic beverages.

Vaccines. Thimerosal is the mercury-containing preservative used in many vaccines. It has also been used in contact lens solutions, eye drops, and immunoglobulins. Additionally it is used in patch testing for people who have dermatitis, conjunctivitis, and other potentially allergic reactions. The body uses selenium to stabilize mercury in the body and keep it from doing damage. Similar to the story with halogens and iodine, mercury uses up this valuable nutrient, as well as causing various other problems.

Electromagnetic fields (EMFs). EMFs are everywhere in our modern world—microwave, cell phone, alarm clock, computer, electrical cables, and the list goes on and on. They all emit electromagnetic waves, which are known to penetrate and influence the body. The thyroid may be among the most sensitive organs to EMF radiation. A study described in the July 2005 *Toxicology Letters* shows just how sensitive the thyroid is to EMF. In this study researchers looked at the effect of the equivalent EMF dose delivered by a cell phone. The researchers wanted to see how this level of EMF impacted thyroid function. T3, T4, and thyroid-stimulating hormone (TSH) were all decreased a significant degree under the influence of the EMFs.[11]

Many Thyroid Conditions Are Due to Adrenal Gland Problems

It's important to understand that in many cases a malfunctioning thyroid gland isn't the actual cause of the hypothyroid condition. Other areas of the body may be responsible, and while different areas of the body can be affected, in many cases weakened adrenal glands are what lead to the development of low thyroid function.

If a health care professional aims treatment only at the thyroid gland and ignores the adrenals and other areas and factors, there may not be a chance of restoring thyroid or adrenal function back to normal. Just prescribing thyroid medication for the rest of a person's life (or radioactive iodine for those with hyperthyroidism) will not address the root problem. The entire endocrine system, including the adrenal glands, needs to be evaluated.

What Causes Adrenal Fatigue?

Adrenal fatigue often develops over a period of years due to unhealthy lifestyle factors such as poor eating habits, poor sleep patterns, and/or chronic stress, which in turn affects the thyroid. For example, someone who eats a lot of refined foods and sugar will have an imbalance in the hormones insulin and cortisol. Eating poorly can, over time, lead to insulin resistance and eventually diabetes, which usually takes years to develop. The constant secretion of cortisol in response to eating poorly and/or dealing with chronic stress can weaken the adrenal glands and eventually lead to adrenal fatigue.

Similarly, not getting enough sleep can weaken the adrenals. Many people stay up late watching television, surfing the Internet, staying out with friends, working, or studying. They get only five to seven hours of sleep; some even less. This is not enough. Most people need eight hours of sleep; some even more. An occasional short night of sleep is not a problem, but on a regular basis, it can affect cortisol levels and weaken adrenal glands. And not dealing with stress effectively has a similar effect on the adrenal and thyroid glands, weakening both.

Trauma, which can be either physical or emotional in nature, such as a car accident, physical or emotional abuse, the death of a loved one, a divorce, or loss of a job, can trigger this disorder as well. This doesn't mean that such traumas cause the immediate development of adrenal fatigue or thyroid problems, but they can be the trigger that over time leads to its development.

When the adrenal glands are weakened, it puts the body in a state of catabolism—the body begins breaking down. When the body is in a catabolic state, the thyroid gland will slow down (become hypothyroid) in an attempt to conserve energy and prevent the body from breaking down more. This makes sense, in that hypothyroidism slows down the metabolism.

There is no magic bullet or supplement that can quickly cure these conditions. But by changing your lifestyle, you can heal these glands and restore your health. It usually doesn't take too long before you start feeling better, and symptoms should lessen within a few weeks if you strictly adhere to a carefully planned juice and living foods regimen. It will take time, though, to completely heal. It's very important to remember that when you start feeling a little better, you should not abandon your healthy lifestyle program.

Adrenal Fatigue Followed My Attack

If you read chapter 1, you know that I was attacked in the night by a burglar while I was house sitting for friends. Following the attack, I suffered extreme adrenal fatigue. I was so tired I could barely drag myself through a day. It felt as if I had a ball and chain wrapped around my body. Just getting dressed in the morning was a huge effort. I remember sitting on the floor in the corner of my bedroom thinking that I was so tired I couldn't get up off the floor. Life was so painful and difficult that it didn't seem worth it to go on. I remember thinking I could go deep inside my soul where there was peace and hide. But I recalled something about a catatonic state (one of near unconsciousness often brought on by shock) from psychology 101. My professor had mentioned that it was hard to bring people out of that state. I thought I'd better not go there just in case I would not want to be there some day. I decided to hang on for just one more day, albeit by a thin thread of hope that things might improve. Obviously, they did.

I looked at my picture on my website the other day. It didn't seem possible that the healthy person I was looking at was the same person who once sat in that room one thought away from "checking out" for good.

Healing the adrenals, indeed the entire body, takes work. It takes the best nutrition you can possibly eat and drink, with a lot of that being live foods rich in biophotons that give life to your body. It takes nutritional supplements of superior quality, along with prayer and intense emotional work.

You can restore burned-out adrenals that are so exhausted they're barely producing cortisol. You can heal your body that feels too tired to move. I know you can. If I could do it, so can you. We're not all that different, you and I. So go for it! Give it all you have. One day, my friend, you'll be standing in your dream as well, just as I'm standing in mine.

Adrenal disease, endocrine imbalances, and thyroid diseases are too prevalent to ignore, especially because of their connection to autoimmune disorders. In our high-stress, highly toxic environment, nobody can afford to ignore information that can prevent or eliminate this insidious thief of energy and vitality.

Read on to discover what you can do to restore the healthy balance and effective function of your whole endocrine system, especially your thyroid gland.

LIFESTYLE FACTORS THAT MAY CONTRIBUTE TO ADRENAL FATIGUE

- Lack of sleep
- Poor food choices (white flour, low fiber, sugar, too few vegetables and fruit, lack of raw food)
- Using sweet or salty food and sweetened or caffeinated drinks as stimulants when tired

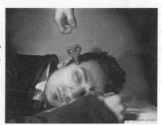

- Staying up late, even though tired
- Feeling or acting powerless
- Continually driving yourself
- Striving to be perfect
- Staying in double binds—no-win situations
- Too few enjoyable and rejuvenating activities
- Trauma, loss, shock, extreme disappointment

3

GETTING BACK TO BETTER THAN NORMAL

Most Americans live a suboptimal existence—mediocre health, low energy, depression, lack of joy, poor memory, poor sleep, and a variety of aches, pains, and ailments. Good health and joyous living are your birthright. You can move toward this quality of life every day if you choose the right lifestyle, which will improve your basal metabolic rate and make it possible for you to have all the energy you need.

As the Juice Lady, I have developed lifestyle guidelines that include a fundamental diet based on juices, smoothies, and living foods. Here's how a "juice and living foods day" might look: Drink two 12- to 16-ounce glasses of raw vegetable juice, or make one glass of juice and have a green smoothie, preferably one in the morning to get you energized and one in the afternoon to keep you going. Eat one or two large salads or servings of raw veggies or a raw energy soup. You could choose a piece of low-sugar raw fruit or some raw veggies for a snack. To that you can add about a quarter of your food cooked.

If you have thyroid problems or another illness or disease, then it is recommended that a larger percentage of your food should be raw (juiced or blended if you have significant digestive issues) and that you occasionally spend a day or two just drinking fresh vegetable juice (juice fasting) to help detoxify your system.

Have you noticed that when you have a day when you eat mostly cooked foods, with very little live food, you want to eat more and more? I experienced that recently. I was served mostly cooked foods at two different events in one day—all whole foods, but about 90 percent of it cooked. At the end of the day I was still hungry. It was 9:00 p.m., and I wanted something else to eat. My body was craving live foods. A little glass of juice did the trick—the urge inside was gone. This is where fresh vegetable juice is so amazing. It's very satisfying. When you feast on raw juices, you can experience the single most effective short-term antidote to cravings, fatigue, and stress available.

Many people call or e-mail to say they feel so much better since they have started on the Juice Lady's living foods lifestyle. I recently received a call from a woman who said those exact words. She has noticed a tremendous amount of energy since starting the living foods and juice program a week before. Prior to that, there were times when she didn't even want to leave the house for days because she was so fatigued. Now she feels like getting out and doing things all the time.

Almost Miraculous

How can such a simple thing make such a huge difference?

Raw juices and living foods are packed with a cornucopia of nutrients, including biophotons—those light rays of energy the plants get from the sun. When we cook food, those beautiful rays of energy are destroyed or shrink way down. Two researchers have found that the light energy in biophotons is an important aspect of food. The more light a food is able to store, the more beneficial the food. Naturally grown fruits and vegetables that are ripened in the sun are strong sources of light energy. Numerous minute particles of light—biophotons, the smallest units of light—make their way into our cells when we eat these foods. They provide our bodies with important information and control complex processes such as ordering and regulating our cells.[1] When you drink a tall glass of fresh veggie juice and your day is focused on more live foods than cooked or processed fare, your whole internal environment changes. As you consume more living foods, you require fewer calories because biophotons help rev up the mitochondria of your cells—the little energy furnaces that pump out ATP (adenosine triphosphate, the energy that is used by cells). They also feed your DNA, which stores about 90 percent of the biophotons found in your cells. Because biophotons carry biological information of the plant into your body, it's kind of like getting a software download or having a computer technician take over your computer remotely to fix things you can't begin to correct. Just as the computer tech fixes errors on your computer, the biophotons help to fix errors that have taken place within the body.[2]

Voilà! You start feeling better, lighter, and more energized as time goes on. Your sleep improves, and you may need less of it. Your mind becomes more alert and creative. No longer will you find yourself in a disorganized fog because biophotons help your mind and body to come alive. You will experience more mental energy, and your creativity improves as well because of the electrical stimulation of the biophotons. (Could this be the boot for dementia or early Alzheimer's disease?)

Your metabolism also ramps up, and you burn more calories, which helps you get fit with greater ease. And in the process, your overall health improves. Symptoms of poor health, ailments, and chronic diseases begin to heal. Your whole life changes!

Live to Your Full Potential

When we eat live foods, our entire bio-terrain operates in peak performance. *Biological terrain* is the system of a cell plus the surrounding environment. It's comprised of fluids, vitamins, minerals, trace elements, enzymes, waste, and microorganisms. When our internal environment becomes overloaded with toxins, waste, and pathogens such as fungi, molds, viruses, or bacteria, when it is deficient in essential nutrients or is too acidic or too alkaline, our cells' vitality is diminished and our immune system is overworked. Then we become susceptible to fatigue, ailments, and diseases.

Raw foods and juices cleanse the body of stored wastes and toxins, which interfere with the proper functioning of the cells, glands, and organs. They provide an abundance of vitamins, minerals, enzymes, phytonutrients, biophotons, and antioxidants that increase the micro-electric potential of each cell. This improves the body's use of oxygen so the muscles and brain are energized. A healthy, vibrant bio-terrain is fundamental to optimal health. This allows our cells, organs, and systems the best chance to do the jobs they were designed to do. A living foods lifestyle can help you achieve this vibrant interior. With a healthy biochemistry, our bodies can deal with stress and challenges far more effectively. It is only when we put congesting, nutrient-depleted, toxic food into our bodies that we tear them down and promote disease. A living foods diet leads to healing and vibrant health.

Do you ever feel like you're just going through the motions of life, existing rather than living out your dreams and purpose?

That can change. You can be so supercharged with health that you live a life of joy and have clarity of mind, and peace of soul. When you care for your body well with the kind of diet recommended in this book, you will have emotional stability and a stronger immune system. You'll be able to deal with stress better than ever before because your nerves won't be on edge with caffeine and sugar. And your willpower will strengthen—a weak body often equates to a weak will.

It may seem too simplistic to say that what you eat could have such a profound impact on your health. Owners of thoroughbred racehorses know the importance of a superior diet—good hay and quality grains, including oats, mineral salts, and vitamins. You wouldn't catch a racehorse owner giving a horse even one little "treat" of bad food, if they're smart.

We're not that different from racehorses. If we want to win the races of our lives, we need a great diet—one that provides quality and energy, one that will take us to the end of our course.

There's also the Seahawks. Chef Mac McNabb says his organic power meals have played a role in the team's success. He doesn't have to be concerned about the price of a salmon entrée and profit margins. "It's all organic and premium meat—grass-fed beef, free-range chicken—and few if any genetically modified foods," *Seattle Times* reported. No sodas or junk food. There aren't any deep-fried foods made in this kitchen—even french fries are baked. For post-practice, when the chef puts out a pasta station, many players will choose something lighter. The days of players such as former defensive tackle Chad Eaton eating three 22-ounce porterhouse steaks in one sitting are rare. This team is eating to win.[3]

How about you? What are you eating for?

How to Achieve a Good Weight With Hypothyroidism

People with an underactive thyroid (hypothyroidism) tend to have a very low basal metabolic rate. One of the most noticeable symptoms of low thyroid is weight gain and difficulty losing weight. Sometimes an overactive thyroid can mimic an underactive one by causing weight gain, but this is less common. For people with low thyroid who are dieting, their metabolism continues to slow down as calories are reduced. That's why some people with low thyroid can have weight gain even when they severely restrict their calories.

More women than men suffer from a sluggish thyroid, or hypothyroidism, and many more women than men with thyroid issues have problems with weight gain. Most thyroid problems occur within the gland itself, but it often isn't discovered until other hormonal imbalances develop. Often thyroid issues, menopause, and weight gain appear together.

Thyroid problems develop in women more than men because:

- Often women spend a lot of their lives dieting, usually in a yo-yo pattern of excess eating and strict fasting. This undermines the metabolism and decreases the metabolic rate, a multipart factor impacting the thyroid, especially during perimenopause.

- Women more than men tend to internalize stress, which affects the adrenal and thyroid glands. Overactive adrenal glands produce excess cortisol, which interferes with thyroid hormones and deposits fat around the midsection. In addition, fatigue caused by overstressed adrenals increases cravings for sweets

and refined carbohydrates to provide quick energy
and feel-good hormones.

- Women's bodies require a delicate balance of hormones such as estrogen and progesterone. These can
be upset when the body is stressed, when it is slightly
acidic, or when it is not getting enough nutritional
support. This results in hormonal imbalances, which
act as a trigger for thyroid problems.

There are a number of symptoms that can be experienced
when you have an underactive thyroid, such as fatigue, depression, weight gain, cold hands and feet, low body temperature,
sensitivity to cold, a feeling of always being chilled, joint pain,
headaches, menstrual disorders, insomnia, dry skin, puffy eyes,
hair loss, brittle nails, constipation, mental dullness, frequent
infections, hoarse voice, ringing in the ears, dizziness, and low
sex drive. If you suspect that you have low thyroid, you should
get tested. Always be aware that you may not test as hypothyroid,
yet you may still have an underactive thyroid gland.

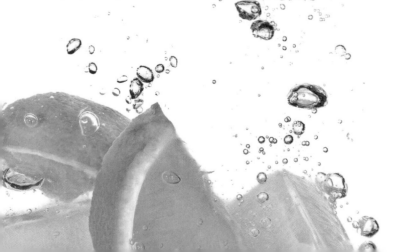

WHAT YOU DON'T KNOW MAY BE KILLING YOUR THYROID

THERE ARE MANY causes of hyperthyroidism (overactive thyroid) and hypothyroidism (underactive thyroid) that are never addressed or treated when diagnosed: things such as imbalances in stress hormones or sex hormones, environmental toxins, food allergies, nutritional deficiencies, inflammation, and infections—all of which may be a source of the problem. Also, poor diet can harm the thyroid's ability to make T4 thyroid hormone as well as the cells' ability to convert T4 into the active form T3.

By understanding some of the major contributing factors in hyper- and hypothyroidism, it is possible to correct the problem and heal this gland.

Psychological factors

Not only are we affected by stress, but we're also affected by our responses to the stressors. Actually, our responses are more important because they determine the degree to which our body is impacted by the stress. Personality issues are also important, such as being high-strung, extremely ambitious, aggressive, or angry responses, which creates more stress.

Dietary factors

You can get too much of a good thing. People who consume too many sea vegetables, iodized salt, stimulants such as caffeine and sodas, or take too much tyrosine may experience hyperthyroidism. On the other hand, excessive consumption of raw cruciferous vegetables (arugula, broccoli, brussels sprouts, cabbage, collard greens, cauliflower, kale, mustard greens, bok choy, radish, horseradish, kohlrabi, turnip, rutabaga, watercress, and rapini) and the mint family (basil, bugleweed, catnip, lavender, lemon balm, marjoram, motherwort, oregano, peppermint, rosemary, spearmint, thyme) can suppress the thyroid gland because they block iodine absorption. This can contribute to hypothyroidism.

All these vegetables and herbs are very good for you, however, and should not be eliminated from your diet but rather rotated with other vegetables. The cruciferous vegetables should be eaten in smaller amounts. (The herbs are not of concern because they're usually eaten in small amounts.) Cooking can help to deactivate some of the goitrogenic compounds in the vegetables and herbs (the compounds that block iodine absorption). Also, soy products (edamame, tofu, tempeh, soy sauce, miso, soy cheese, soymilk, textured vegetable protein) and peanuts are in the same category (goitrogenic) and block iodine absorption. Additionally, deficiencies of iodine, zinc, and vitamins A, B_2, B_3, B_6, and E can contribute to hypothyroidism.

ARE NONSTICK PANS AFFECTING YOUR THYROID?

Ryan Robbins, ND, a naturopathic physician and resident at Bastyr Center for Natural Health, posted an article on Bastyr's website in which he stated,

"For several years, synthetic chemicals have been suspected of contributing to thyroid conditions such as hypo- and hyperthyroidism, as well as thyroid cancer. In the United States, 16 percent of women and 3 percent of men will develop some form of thyroid disease during their lives." [1]

Robbins explains that one group of chemicals—perfluorinated compounds (PFCs)—causes great concern. They are used to make nonstick cookware. They're also used in stain-resistant carpeting, rugs, and fabrics; flame-resistant and waterproof clothing; wood sealants; paints; and food packaging.

Two of these PFCs—perfluorooctane sulfonate (PFOS) and perfluorooctanoic acid (PFOA)—cause cancer and lead to hormone disruption and liver damage, according to Robbins. And according to a 2010 report in the journal Environmental Health Perspectives, men and women with high PFOA levels were twice as likely to have a thyroid disorder as those with lower levels. [2]

To avoid exposure to these chemicals, here is what Robbins recommends:

- Eat only whole food and avoid all packaged, processed foods.
- Avoid slick food packaging such as microwave popcorn bags and coated coffee cups.
- Use only stainless steel, glass, or ceramic mugs and stainless water bottles for all drinks, but especially for hot drinks; avoid plastic and Styrofoam cups. Tote your food in reusable glass or ceramic ware.

- Use safer alternatives to Teflon such as Thermolon (used in Green Pan cookware), seasoned cast iron, or glass cookware. It's best not to use Teflon at all; when it's heated to 260 degrees, it starts releasing toxic gases into the air we breathe.

- Use only natural cleaning products such as baking soda, white vinegar, and vegetable oil-based soaps.

- Avoid all stain-resistant carpeting, rugs, and fabrics, and all fire-retardant and waterproof fabrics, mattresses, and clothing.

- Drink only purified water that has had toxic organic compounds removed.[3]

What to Avoid

Sugar of all types

Sweeteners can be a big problem for the thyroid gland. Sugar can cause "burnout" for both the thyroid and adrenal glands. Blood sugar changes can also promote diabetes and hypoglycemia, both of which often occur in people with thyroid issues. Some people report increased energy and that their thyroid levels stabilize when they stop eating sweets altogether. Sweets also cause a rise in triglycerides, so avoiding them can help return triglycerides to a normal level.

Goitrogens

Goitrogens are substances that suppress the function of the thyroid gland by interfering with iodine uptake. Following are the goitrogenic foods you should avoid or greatly reduce.

Soy. Soy is one of the most prevalent goitrogens

(iodine-blockers). The National Center for Toxicological Research showed that the isoflavones in soy are damaging to the thyroid in adults and especially worrisome in children because they block thyroid peroxidase.[4]

Soy contains estrogenic compounds that can interfere with thyroid hormones and sex hormones, contributing to PMS, cramps, bloating, and menopause symptoms. Some people with hyperactive thyroid find that small amounts of soy (organic only, because soy is a big GMO crop) help modulate their thyroid gland. But people with low thyroid should avoid soy altogether—no tofu, textured vegetable protein, soymilk, soy cheese, soy ice cream, tempeh, seitan, miso, or edamame.[5]

One retrospective epidemiological study showed that teenaged children with autoimmune thyroid disease were more likely to have received soy formula as infants (eighteen out of fifty-nine children; 31 percent) compared to healthy siblings (nine out of seventy-six; 12 percent) or control group children (seven out of fifty-four; 13 percent).[6]

Watch out for soybean oil in salad dressings, mayonnaise, and snack foods; also textured vegetable protein, which is soy. It's used as filler in a lot of snack foods and energy bars. Use almond, oat, hemp, or rice milk instead of soy milk. And avoid soy ice cream, soy cheese, and soy protein powder.

Cruciferous vegetables. A family of vegetables known as the cruciferous or mustard family contains goitrogenic chemicals that suppress the thyroid. Some goitrogenic compounds induce antibodies that cross-react with the thyroid gland; others interfere with thyroid peroxidase (TPO), the enzyme responsible for adding iodine while thyroid hormones are produced. Like isoflavones in soy, isothiocyanates in cruciferous veggies appear to reduce thyroid function by blocking TPO. These vegetables include broccoli, cauliflower, spinach, kale, mustard, brussels sprouts, cabbage, bok choy, turnips, rutabagas, radish, horse-radish, arugula, rapini, canola, and kohlrabi. Foods and herbs from the cruciferous and mint families are very nutritious, and many have important medicinal properties. Regular consumption of these plants will not lead to underactive thyroid function unless other factors are also involved, particularly iodine deficiency.

Only those who already have hypothyroidism need to be concerned. In these cases, foods from the cruciferous family should be reduced but not eliminated from the diet. Cooking does appear to help deactivate the goitrogenic compounds found in these vegetables. As I stated earlier, spices and herbs from the mint family aren't as much of a concern because they aren't consumed in as large a quantity. However, regular consumption of herbal products containing bugleweed, motherwort, and lemon balm should be avoided.

Other goitrogenic foods that lower thyroid function include peanuts, peanut butter, and millet.

Polyunsaturated oils

These oils include soy, corn, safflower, sunflower, and cotton-seed. They interfere with thyroid gland function and the response of tissues to thyroid hormone because these longer-chain fatty acids are deposited in cells more often as rancid, oxidized fat. Oxidized oils block thyroid hormone secretions. This impairs the body's ability to convert T4 to T3, which creates the enzymes needed to convert fats to energy. When this breakdown occurs, one can develop symptoms typical of hypothyroidism. Try virgin coconut oil instead. It does not oxidize and turn rancid easily.

Food allergens

When it comes to food-related allergies that impact the thyroid gland, it is not like eating a nut or a shrimp and getting an immediate reaction. The type of reaction that disrupts thyroid function is a delayed interaction with food antigens that can occur up to four days after eating the food.

The two most prevalent food-related reactions come from dairy and wheat. These two foods are known in alternative medicine to be highly correlated with autoimmune thyroiditis. Dairy and wheat gluten are often removed from diets of thyroid patients with good success. The *Journal of Clinical Gastroenterology* demonstrated that those allergic to gluten had a much greater risk of thyroid abnormalities.[7]

Gluten and casein

Go gluten and casein free. Today's most common allergies and food intolerances are from wheat and dairy products due to the hybridized proteins of gluten and a1 casein. These proteins can cause "leaky gut," which in turn will cause inflammation of the thyroid and affect its function. Follow a grain-free diet if possible or at least go gluten free. Only consume dairy products that come from goat milk or sheep milk. Several studies show a strong link between Hashimoto's and Graves' Disease and gluten intolerance. Chris Kessler, a recognized leader in ancestral health, Paleo nutrition, and functional and integrative medicine, explains that the molecular structure of gliadin, the protein in gluten, closely resembles that of the thyroid gland. When gliadin leaks beyond the protective barrier of the gut and enters the bloodstream, the immune system attacks it. The antibodies to gliadin also cause the body to attack thyroid tissue. This means if you have autoimmune thyroid disease (AITD) and you consume foods containing gluten, your immune system will attack your thyroid.[8] Think you can splurge on gluten-containing bread, pasta, or pizza once in a while? Unfortunately the immune response to gluten can last up to six months each time you eat it. This is why it is critical to eliminate gluten completely from your diet...forever...if you have AITD.[9]

Gluten intolerance research pioneer Dr. Kenneth Fine has found that one in three Americans are gluten intolerant. Kressler says, "Gluten intolerance can also present with inflammation in the joints, skin, respiratory tract, and brain—without any obvious gut symptoms." How do you know if you are gluten intolerant? You could get a stool test. But if you have gluten intolerance, your test for gluten antibodies may be falsely negative if you have Th1-dominant Hashimoto's. There can also be other problems with the testing that cause gluten intolerance not to show up. That is why it's best to just eat gluten free. He explained that foods that contain gluten (both whole grains and flours) contain substances that inhibit nutrient absorption, damage the intestinal lining, and activate a potentially destructive autoimmune response.[10]

Some carbohydrates

Lower carbohydrate intake—lower your intake of grains (a major source of carbs) and replace them with plenty of vegetables, clean proteins, and healthy fats. Most women especially consume far too many carbs, which increase estrogen and negatively affect the thyroid. Instead consume healthy fats that will balance hormones, such as coconut oil, coconut milk, avocado, grass-fed beef, wild salmon, chia, flaxseeds, and hemp seeds.

Iodized salt

Replace iodized salt with Celtic sea salt because table salt is a problem for some people with thyroid challenges. Also, choose only natural sources of iodine.

Halogens: chlorine, fluoride, and bromine

Halogens (fluorine, chlorine, bromine, and astatine) are now becoming ubiquitous in our environment and have major consequences for thyroid function. Since iodine shares chemical properties with other halogens such as chlorine, fluorine, and bromine, these halogens can displace iodine and disrupt thyroid function. Chlorine is added to our municipal water supply.

Fluoride will impede the absorption of iodine. Fluoride is added to city water treatment all across America. Unless you have a special water purification system that takes out fluoride, you will be drinking it. It's added to toothpaste, so you will need to shop for fluoride-free toothpaste. And avoid getting your teeth painted with fluoride at the dental office.

Many popular sports and electrolyte drinks contain brominated vegetable oil. Bromine also is used in some baked goods and fire-retardant compounds. Bromine-based fire retardants used in carpets, mattresses, upholstery, furniture, and various electronic equipment have become suspect for causing or contributing to hypothyroidism.[11]

A study published in *Physiological Research* showed that bromine intake blocks iodine uptake by the thyroid and increases its excretion through the urine.[12]

Bromism, a condition of excess bromine intake, is known to have drastic effects on the nervous system—a situation common among low-thyroid sufferers. Based on research, bromides have also been linked to behavioral problems, neurodevelopmental delays, and attention-deficit hyperactivity disorder (ADD/ADHD) in children.

Splenda (sucralose) is made when hydroxyl groups in a sugar molecule are replaced with chlorine molecules—the same chlorine atoms used to disinfect swimming pools. We know that polychlorinated biphenyls and organochlorines from pesticides and other sources alter thyroid function and impede weight loss. The journal *Obesity Reviews* highlights the effect chlorine molecules have on thyroid and weight loss. This article shows that chlorine molecules that accumulate in human fat tissue are released during weight loss and impair thyroid function, potentially leading to weight-loss resistance.[13]

Based on this research, the fact that Splenda, which contains artificially placed chlorine molecules, is marketed as a "diet sweetener" seems to be an oxymoron of advertising.

But thyroid problems and weight-loss resistance are not the only concerns with this product. We do not know the long-term health effects that Splenda will have on the human body because it's a relatively new product, but the Food and Drug Administration (FDA) has given a review of possible side effects from consuming this artificial sweetener, including enlarged liver and kidneys, decreased white blood cell count, reduced growth rate, and decreased fetal body weight.[14]

I recommend that you completely avoid this sweetener.

Mercury

Mercury is a toxic metal that can significantly impact the thyroid. There is ample evidence that mercury leaches from dental amalgam fillings and contributes to thyroid disease and anemia along with a host of other physical problems. While large doses of mercury can induce hyperthyroidism, smaller amounts can induce hypothyroidism by interfering with both the production of thyroxine (T4) and the conversion of T4 to T3. Mercury also disturbs the metabolism of copper and zinc, which are two minerals critical to thyroid function. Gray hair can be an indication of mercury accumulation, more so in women than men.

Mercury can cause disruptions to the immune system and it promotes the production of antibodies produced by the immune system, which also are involved in autoimmune thyroid disease. There are different forms of mercury—organic and inorganic—that can have different effects on the thyroid. It is believed that estrogen and milk can cause an increase in the absorption of mercury. Mercury also hinders the availability of selenium-dependent enzymes. These are the same enzymes used by the thyroid to make thyroid hormone.

LOW THYROID LINKED TO HIGH CHOLESTEROL[15]

When your thyroid gland doesn't produce enough hormone, metabolism can slow, having a direct impact on the body's ability to clear cholesterol from the bloodstream. This means that the risk of heart disease can increase as cholesterol builds up in the arteries, especially around the heart. This buildup of cholesterol can make it difficult for your heart to pump efficiently. This is why hypothyroidism can sometimes lead to an enlarged heart and heart failure.

According to studies by the University of Texas-Southwest Medical School, Dallas, Texas, there is a clear correlation between hypothyroidism and high blood cholesterol. They found that 90 percent of those with overt hypothyroidism also have increased cholesterol and/or triglycerides. "Once hypothyroidism is treated," they reported, "and the TSH level is restored to normal, the majority of patients show an estimated 20 to 30 percent reduction in cholesterol levels."

The Mayo Clinic states that "hypothyroidism may also be associated with an increased risk of heart disease, primarily because high levels of low-density lipoprotein (LDL) cholesterol—the 'bad' cholesterol—can occur in people with an underactive thyroid. It is not unusual when low thyroid function is addressed, cholesterol will often return to normal levels."

NOURISH YOUR THYROID WITH LIVING FOODS

L IVING FOODS. THEY'RE foods that are alive—raw (not cooked) and filled with life. They're also called raw foods or live foods. You can plant them, pick them, sprout them, or simply eat them. In each case—you get life! That's because life comes from life. These foods are your "true north," your path home to health in a jungle of dietary havoc, contaminated food, and abounding confusion about what and how to eat.

Good health is the result of consuming whole, unprocessed, clean food with a large percentage of that being raw and alive. These foods are chock-full of nutrients, water, and fiber that flush away toxins, waste, and "sludge" from our cells and intercellular fluids. They help us prevent disease. They alkalize our bodies and help us restore our pH balance. And they give our cells vital light rays of energy to help them communicate more effectively.

Living Foods Every Day of Your Life

I have created a program that involves juicing every day and eating a large percentage of your food while it is still "living," which means uncooked and unprocessed plant foods. These living foods "love you back" by giving you a plethora of life-giving nutrients. That equates to higher energy levels, weight loss, detoxification, mental clarity, increased vitality, and inner peace.

But unlike most raw food programs, the Juice Lady's living foods lifestyle program doesn't toss out all cooked food. You can even include a few organic, pastured animal products if you wish. This lifestyle is about choosing pure, whole foods with an abundance of that fare being live—raw, juiced, blended, gently warmed, and dehydrated.

Raw green vegetables are emphasized because they have served as the basis of nearly all life on this planet. They're key to our life. I've known this for a long time, but I couldn't get enough of them into my diet to really make a big difference—until I started juicing about a quart a day that included lots of greens. I rotated a wide variety of greens such as Swiss chard, collards, curly kale, black dino kale, kohlrabi leaves, dandelion greens, romaine lettuce, parsley, and spinach, combined with cucumber, celery, lemon, and a carrot or two.

Juicing this wide variety of produce provides a powerhouse of vitamins, minerals, enzymes, phytonutrients, and biophotons. These foods help to lower estrogen in a woman's body and decrease the chance of contracting breast cancer—something I've always been concerned about since my mother died of breast cancer when I was six years old. Raw foods, which are rich in antioxidants, also help the body remove toxins, thus helping to prevent illnesses.

Any diet that is made up of 60 to 80 percent raw foods is a live foods diet, because the majority of foods are eaten in their natural state. Living foods are high in enzymes, which are important to the body because they help in converting vitamins and minerals to energy. Indeed, enzymes are needed for every chemical reaction that takes place in the body. No mineral, vitamin, or hormone can do its work without enzymes. Plant food enzymes work in the digestive system where they predigest foods and thus spare the pancreas and other digestive organs from having to work so hard to produce excess enzymes. Eating living foods, especially vegetables, sprouts, wild greens, fruits, nuts, and seeds, is the healthiest for the human body. Truly they can transform you from the inside out.

Living Foods for Thyroid Health

Since your thyroid is a key gland that's tied to every other system in your body, it needs to work flawlessly. When it's out of balance, you're out of balance. If you have a number of the symptoms of low thyroid, as indicated by the Low Thyroid Health Quiz in chapter 2, chances are that you could benefit by working on your thyroid health by eating more living foods.

Some foods boost thyroid function, which makes them perfect for treating hypothyroidism, while others suppress thyroid function, which can help people with hyperthyroidism. And there are certain foods that are best avoided by anyone who is concerned about having a healthy thyroid gland and overall good health.

The following raw foods are among the most helpful for restoring thyroid balance whether you have an underactive or overactive thyroid:

- Fresh raw vegetable juices
- Low-sugar fruit, especially lemons, limes, cranberries and other berries, and green apples
- Raw nuts and seeds
- Seaweed for its rich iodine content (for hypothyroid)
- Chlorophyll-rich green juices such as watercress, collards, chard, kale, kohlrabi leaves, beet greens, and parsley (vary the cruciferous greens with other

non-cruciferous greens, such as lettuce, beet greens, watercress, and spinach, if you have hypothyroidism)

Food Solutions for Those With Hypothyroidism

Making dietary changes is your first line of defense in treating low thyroid. Many people with hypothyroidism experience crippling fatigue and brain fog, which prompts them to reach for quick forms of energy such as sugar and caffeine. These two unhealthy substances can burn out your thyroid and destabilize blood sugar faster than anything else.

When I did my internship with a nutritional MD, he'd always say, "Caffeine and sugar are to the thyroid and adrenals like whipping a poor tired horse that just wants to rest." Stay away from sugar and caffeine; they can cause the overproduction of stress hormones—namely adrenaline and cortisol—that can hinder thyroid function and further burn out your thyroid.

In order to fix your metabolism, you need to nourish your thyroid gland, remove the foods and substances that suppress it, and work on your overall health. Here's what you can do:

- Consume plenty of iodine-rich foods, including fish, seafood, sea vegetables, eggs, cranberries, spinach, and green bell peppers.

- Increase your protein. Protein transports thyroid hormone to all your tissues, so enjoy it at each meal. Proteins include nuts and nut butters; quinoa; hormone- and antibiotic-free animal products (organic, grass-fed meats, eggs, and sustainably-farmed fish); and legumes (beans, lentils, dried peas).

- Use Celtic sea salt; avoid iodized sodium chloride (table salt). Celtic sea salt naturally contains iodine with a full complement of minerals that work together.

- Take a good multivitamin-mineral supplement.

- Get fat into your diet. Fat is your friend. Cholesterol is the precursor to hormonal pathways. If you consume insufficient fat and cholesterol, you could be exacerbating hormonal imbalances, including thyroid hormones. Healthy fats include olive oil; ghee; avocados; flax seeds; fish; nuts and nut butters; and virgin coconut oil.

- Use virgin coconut oil in food preparation. Polyunsaturated oils such as soy, corn, safflower, and sunflower oil are damaging to the thyroid gland because they oxidize quickly and become rancid. The opposite effect happens with virgin coconut oil; it does not oxidize and turn rancid easily.

- Cranberries are an excellent low-sugar fruit. Buy them in the fall and freeze some for when they're out of season. They contain iodine, which is good for the thyroid.

THERMOGENIC FOODS REV UP YOUR METABOLISM

Thermogenesis means the production of heat, which raises metabolism and burns calories. Thermogenic foods are essentially fat-burning foods and spices that help increase your fat-burning potential just by eating them. Include these foods often in your juices:

Hot peppers—One study found that the animals studied developed obesity mainly because they didn't produce enough heat after eating, not because the animals ate more or were less active.[1] Another study found that hot peppers turn up the internal heat, which helps in burning calories.[2] You can add hot peppers or a dash of hot sauce to many juice recipes and they'll taste delicious.

Garlic—Garlic is a good source of selenium. Deficiencies of iodine and selenium are implicated in hypothyroidism. Garlic is also a known appetite suppressant; the strong odor of garlic stimulates the satiety center in the brain, thereby reducing feelings of hunger. It also increases the brain's sensitivity to leptin, a hormone produced by fat cells that regulates appetite.

Ginger—Ginger root is a great source of zinc, which is needed for the hypothalamus to stimulate the pituitary gland to signal the thyroid gland to produce thyroid hormone. Ginger also contains a substance that stimulates gastric enzymes, which can boost metabolism, and it has been shown to be an anti-inflammatory.

It helps improve gastric motility—the spontaneous peristaltic movements of the stomach that aid in moving food through the digestive system. It has also been found to lower cholesterol. It tastes delicious in juice recipes; I add it to almost every juice recipe I make.

More Food Choices to Help Your Body Heal

Though I recommend that you always buy organically grown produce, it is especially important for thyroid sufferers to avoid conventionally grown foods on the "dirty dozen" list.

THE DIRTY DOZEN LIST[3]

- Apples
- Celery
- Cherry tomatoes
- Cucumbers
- Grapes
- Hot peppers
- Nectarines (imported)
- Peaches
- Potatoes
- Spinach
- Strawberries
- Bell peppers

THE CLEANEST FOODS LIST[4]

- Asparagus
- Avocados
- Cabbage
- Cantaloupe
- Cauliflower
- Sweet corn (no GMO corn)
- Eggplant
- Grapefruit
- Kiwi
- Mangoes
- Onions
- Papaya
- Pineapple
- Sweet peas (frozen)
- Sweet potatoes

Simple Living Foods Meal Plan for Stressed Adrenals and Thyroid

In chapter 2 I described the connection between adrenal fatigue and thyroid problems. Here is a sample diet plan that can help restore stressed adrenals as well as your thyroid function:

Sample diet plan (Day 1)

Upon rising

Start your day with ⅛ to ½ teaspoon of Celtic sea salt or kelp powder dissolved in a glass of water, juice, or herbal tea. Drink another glass at your lowest energy point during the day. When the adrenal glands are fatigued, they do not produce enough aldosterone. Aldosterone regulates the amount of sodium and potassium in the body. When aldosterone becomes deficient, not enough salt is retained in the body. Have you been craving salt? This is probably the reason.

Avoid caffeine

Coffee, black tea, and possibly even green tea for a while (although it has ⅓ the caffeine of coffee) should be avoided. Even white tea, which has the least caffeine of all, may be too much for your weak adrenals.

Breakfast

Try the Adrenal Booster Cocktail followed by a Healthy Green Smoothie (see chapter 8).

Midmorning or midafternoon

Have a fresh juice midmorning and/or mid- to late afternoon. Dark green juices are particularly beneficial.

Lunch and dinner

Raw foods are helpful as well for their superior nutrients and biophotons. You can choose raw food recipes, some cooked food recipes, and some animal products that are organic, grass fed, and free range, if you are not a vegan. Eat lots of high-fiber vegetables. There is a need for high-quality protein as well. You may need some animal protein for a while unless you go mostly raw and really focus on getting enough high-quality protein from seeds, nuts, sprouts, and dark leafy greens. You may also need to supplement with free-form amino acids. The amino acid program has made a significant difference for many people I've worked with. Also, keep your blood sugar balanced. Eat smaller meals and a couple of very nutritious snacks during the day.

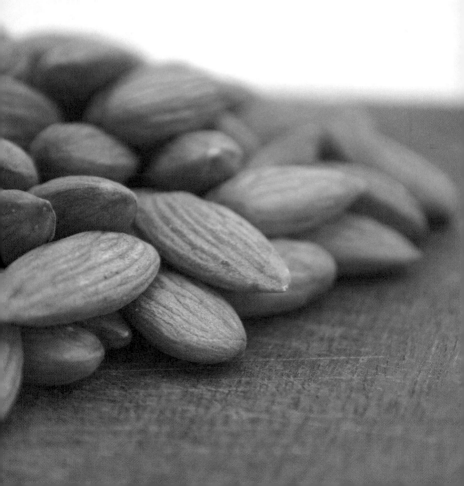

NUTRIENTS THAT SUPPORT THE THYROID

THYROID PROBLEMS CAN develop for many reasons that we've already discovered, such as genetics, stress, environmental factors, and autoimmune disease, but most commonly they come from nutritional deficiencies, specifically iodine and selenium. Hypothyroidism (underactive thyroid) is more common than hyperthyroidism (overactive), which underlines the importance of activating a supply chain of the critical nutrients that are deficient. Not only should you look for prime sources of iodine and selenium, for instance, but as I have mentioned in chapter 4, you must avoid foods that rob your body of those important minerals, or that inhibit them from staying at health-promoting levels.

It is imperative to provide the thyroid gland with all the nutritional cofactors needed to make thyroid hormone. So in this chapter I am going to give you lists of supplements, vitamins, minerals, and herbs that improve thyroid function. Some will come with daily recommended doses, others will come with a short list of foods you can eat to get those nutrients working in your body.

Supplements That Help You Fight Thyroid Disorders

Iodine

Iodine is the most critical nutrient for good thyroid function, so you should consume more iodine-rich foods, such as seaweed and other sea vegetables, seafood and fish, and even cranberries that have been harvested from bogs near a seacoast. You may also want to take supplemental iodine. Lugol's is a popular brand of liquid iodine. Consume more of these iodine-rich foods: sea veggies, kelp, and dulse; seafood and fish; and cranberries (grown in bogs on the coastline; they contain iodine).

Selenium

Selenium may be the "hero" of nutritional supplement thyroid therapies. Many people diagnosed with hypothyroidism have been found to be selenium deficient. Selenium deficiency can reduce the activity of thyroid hormones, because it is essential for converting T4 thyroid hormone into T3. It may also have the ability to suppress anti-thyroid antibodies in people who suffer from thyroid inflammation or thyroiditis. Reversing a selenium deficiency could, in some people, actually repair thyroid metabolism by increasing the intracellular conversion of T4 to T3. Foods rich in selenium include seafood, Brazil nuts, barley, red Swiss chard, oats, brown rice, beef, lamb, turnips, garlic, barley, egg yolk, chicken, radishes, and pecans.

Zinc

Zinc is needed for the hypothalamus to stimulate the pituitary gland, which signals the thyroid gland to produce thyroid hormone. Ginger root is one of the best sources of zinc.

Vitamin D

Vitamin D is particularly important, and most people are deficient. Not only does Vitamin D help transport thyroid hormones into our cells and help contribute to proper hormonal pathways (it's actually a hormone, not a vitamin), it's also an immune modulator, meaning that it can help regulate immune function. Vitamin D is necessary for thyroid hormone production in the pituitary gland and possibly in binding T3 to its receptor. Vitamin D is a critical nutrient that also affects bone health and even cancer prevention. If you haven't been tested, it would be wise to get a blood test and know where your vitamin D levels stand.

Multivitamin

Take a good multivitamin to ensure you're getting the basic nutrients.

Tyrosine

An amino acid, tyrosine is needed by the body to manufacture thyroid hormones from iodine.

Glutathione

A powerful antioxidant that strengthens the immune system, glutathione is one of the pillars of help for the thyroid. It can boost your body's ability to modulate and regulate the immune system, dampen autoimmune flare-ups, and protect and heal thyroid tissue.

Bladderwrack

A type of seaweed that is a rich source of iodine, bladder-wrack is used to stimulate the thyroid gland thus increasing metabolism.

Other Nutrients and What Foods to Juice Daily to Benefit From Them

Vitamin C

2,000–4,000 mg/day with bioflavonoids

Foods to juice: hot peppers, kale, parsley, collards, turnip greens, broccoli, mustard greens, watercress, lemons with white part, and spinach

Vitamin E

800 IU/day with mixed tocopherols

Foods to juice: spinach, asparagus, and carrots

Niacin

125–150 mg/day, as niacinamide

Pyridoxine (vitamin B6)

150 mg/day

Foods to juice: spinach, kale, avocado (green smoothies)

Pantothenic acid (vitamin B$_5$)

1,200–1,500 mg/day

Foods to juice: broccoli, kale

Vitamin B-100 Complex

I suggest B Complex 12; take as directed.

Magnesium citrate

400–1,200 mg/day

Foods to juice: beet greens, spinach, parsley, dandelion greens, garlic, beets, carrots, celery, avocado (green smoothies)

Trace minerals

Multi-minerals; they have a calming effect

I suggest Citramins (multi-minerals); take as directed.

Foods to juice: Dark leafy greens are especially rich in minerals.

Herbs That Promote Healthy Thyroid Function

Rhodiola rosea

Enhances memory and concentration; has been shown to reduce stress-induced fatigue and improve mental performance

Holy basil leaf

Helps to normalize cortisol in times of stress

Wild oats milky seed

Supports the nervous system

Schisandra berry

Helps with energy, endurance, and resistance to stress

Ashwagandha

Has been shown to have a sedating effect on the body and helps to rebuild the digestive and nervous systems

Siberian ginseng

Has been used traditionally to stimulate and nourish the adrenal glands and increases mental alertness

Cordyceps

A Chinese mushroom used for supporting the adrenal gland; can also help the immune function

Licorice root (not the candy)

Provides a lift for the adrenal glands and improves resistance to stress; should be used in small amounts according to directions since it can raise blood pressure when higher quantities are used

Remember, every journey begins with the first step. Once you adopt a juice and living foods diet as part of your new lifestyle, it will take more than a couple of weeks to see a profound difference, although many people report significant improvements in just a few days. Give the juice and living foods lifestyle six months at least and then evaluate. If you haven't noticed profound changes, then you're the first one I've encountered to say that. You should be feeling so much better that you'll never want to go back to your old lifestyle. And you can be on your way to living your potential to the fullest!

Chapter 7

REV UP YOUR METABOLISM WITH FRESH JUICES AND SMOOTHIES

IT IS BELIEVED that our ancient ancestors ate up to six pounds of green leaves per day. Can you imagine eating a grocery bag full of seasonal greens each and every day? Few of us eat even the minimum USDA recommendation of five servings of vegetables and fruit a day or three cups of dark green vegetables per week. And yet, green veggies deliver a bonanza of vitamins, minerals, enzymes, biophotons, and phytonutrients. The good news is that you can juice them and easily consume one to three cups of greens per day.

Calorie for calorie, dark green leafy vegetables are among the most concentrated sources of nutrition. They are a rich source of minerals including iron, calcium, potassium, and magnesium plus vitamins K, C, and E, along with many of the B vitamins. They also provide a variety of phytonutrients including alpha- and beta-carotene, lutein, and zeaxanthin, which protect our cells from damage and our eyes from age-related diseases. Dark green leaves even contain small amounts of omega-3 fats.

Juicing is one way you can get these power-packed beauti-fiers into your diet every day. There are many greens that can be juiced such as collard leaves, chard, beet tops, kale, kohl-rabi leaves, mustard greens, parsley, spinach, lettuce, cilantro, watercress, arugula, and dandelion greens. All you need is a juicer and some great-tasting recipes to make a significant change in your health.

Green juices are good because even if you took the time to chew up a couple of cups of green veggies each day, you wouldn't get as much benefit from them as you would from juicing them up. It's the mechanical process of juicing the vegetables that breaks apart plant-cell walls and makes absorption better than even the best-chewed food. It has an effect like throwing marbles at a chain link fence rather than tennis balls—juiced contents are going to go through your intestinal tract in a way that "tennis ball-size" nutrients can't.

Juice contains easily absorbed micronutrients that will optimize your overall health and wellness. Green juices energize your body, fire up your metabolism, speed weight loss, and overhaul your health.

Not All Green Juices Are Good for Thyroid Disorders

Although I love my green drinks, not all greens are the same. Here's the problem: Most green juices feature kale, spinach, or cruciferous vegetables as the basic ingredient. While many people can drink these juices without any trouble, this is not true for those who are struggling with a thyroid condition (or susceptible to one). If you have a thyroid disorder, you will need to pick and choose your ingredients. Some are extra-helpful for thyroid function, but other kinds of greens are not. True, the latter are only harmful in large quantities or when juiced daily, but many of them are just the kinds of super-veggies that you may want to use on a daily basis. Still, by limiting them and balancing them with other foods and nutrients, you may be able to glean the best from all.

Good—if varied with others—are chlorophyll-rich green juices such as watercress, collards, chard, kale, kohlrabi leaves, beet greens, and parsley. (Vary the cruciferous greens with other non-cruciferous greens, such as lettuce, beet greens, watercress, and spinach, if you have hypothyroidism.) Cruciferous vegetables include the well-known broccoli and cauliflower, kale and brussels sprouts, as well as vegetables less often classed with them such as horseradish, bok choy, cabbage, spinach, mustard greens, turnips, rutabagas, arugula, rapini, and kohlrabi.

The important thing to know is that anyone with a thyroid disorder needs to balance the cruciferous greens (many of which also contain thyroid-enhancing components) with the many other fresh ingredients that are known to aid thyroid function, and to choose non-cruciferous greens much of the time.

Other bitter greens that combine well with vegetables and fruit include:

- Beet greens—purple-red veins and bright green flesh on the leaves; very tangy with a hint of mustard and beet

- Cress—watercress is widely available; the taste is hot, sharp, and biting

- Kale—large deep green leaves, curled at the edges; resembles broccoli in flavor but with a peppery, bitter finish

- Mustards—red or green leaves; sharp, pungent with a hint of hot mustard and horseradish flavor

- Swiss chard—broad, fan-shaped green leaf, wide white stems and veins (some have red or yellow veins); mildly bitter

The reason that cruciferous vegetables are watch-listed for juicers with thyroid disorders is because they are what's called "goitrogens." As I mentioned earlier in chapter 4, goitrogens are substances that suppress the function of the thyroid gland by interfering with iodine uptake. (This can cause an enlargement of the thyroid, otherwise known as a goiter.) Iodine is vital for production of thyroid hormone. Especially for people who already have an underactive thyroid, consuming raw cruciferous veggies can further suppress thyroid hormone creation.

Soy also carries goitrogenic properties, although the goitro-genic isoflavones are disabled in fermented soy products. Smaller amounts of goitrogens can be found in spinach, strawberries, peaches, and peanuts (including peanut butter).

Your goal should not be to eliminate goitrogenic foods alto-gether, because they have so many health-promoting properties, including protection against certain cancers, but to limit them to reasonable daily amounts—or cook them. Cooking cruciferous veggies deactivates the goitrogenic compounds, as their isothio-cyanates appear to be heat-sensitive.

All About Juicing

Whether you are just getting started juicing or you've been juicing a long time, you probably have a few questions about this subject. It's about time to answer them. I hope to inspire you to make juicing a daily habit, whether you want to go green or any other color in the juice rainbow.

Every time you pour yourself a glass of freshly made juice, picture a big vitamin-mineral cocktail with a wealth of nutrients that promote vitality. The veggies are broken down into an easily absorbable form that your body can use right away. This food doesn't have to go through a big process of breaking everything down, so it goes to work in your body to give you energy and renew you right down to your cells. It also spares your organs all the work it takes to digest food, and that equates to more energy. It detoxifies your body as well because it's rich in antioxidants, which lightens your load so that your body doesn't have to work as hard to deal with all the toxic stuff.

In addition to water and easily absorbed protein and carbohydrates, juice also provides essential fatty acids, vitamins, minerals, enzymes, and phytonutrients. And researchers are continuing to explore how the nutrients found in juice help the body heal and shed unwanted pounds.

The next time you make a glass of fresh juice, this is what you'll be drinking:

Protein. Did you ever consider juice to be a source of protein? Surprisingly it does offer more than you might think. We use protein to form muscles, ligaments, tendons, hair, nails, and skin. Protein is needed to create enzymes, which direct chemical reactions, and hormones that guide bodily functions. Fruits and vegetables contain lower quantities of protein than animal foods such as muscle meats and dairy products. Therefore, they are thought of as poor protein sources. But juices are concentrated forms of vegetables and fruit, and so provide easily absorbed amino acids, the building blocks that make up protein. For example, sixteen ounces of carrot juice (two to three pounds of carrots) provides about five grams of protein (the equivalent of about one chicken wing or two ounces of tofu). Vegetable protein is not complete protein so it does not provide all the amino acids your body needs. In addition to lots of dark leafy greens, you'll want to eat other protein sources, such as sprouts, legumes (beans, lentils, and split peas), nuts, seeds, and whole grains. If you're not vegan, you can add eggs, and free-range, grass-fed muscle meats such as chicken, turkey, lamb, and beef along with wild-caught fish.

Carbohydrates. Vegetable juice contains carbohydrates. Carbs provide fuel for the body, which it uses for movement, heat production, and chemical reactions. The chemical bonds of carbohydrates lock in the energy a plant takes up from the sun, and this energy is released when the body burns plant food as fuel. There are three categories of carbs: simple (sugars), complex (starches and fiber), and fiber. Choose more complex carbohydrates in your diet than simple carbs. There are more simple sugars in fruit juice than vegetable juice, which is why you should juice more vegetables and in most cases drink no more than four ounces of fruit juice a day. Both insoluble and soluble fibers are found in whole fruits and vegetables, and both types are needed for good health. Who said juice doesn't have fiber? Juice has the soluble form—pectin and gums, which are excellent for the digestive tract. Soluble fiber also helps to lower blood cholesterol levels, stabilize blood sugar, and improve good bowel bacteria.

Essential fatty acids. There is very little fat in fruit and vegetable juices, but the fats juice does contain are essential to your health. The essential fatty acids (EFAs)—linoleic and alpha-linolenic acids in particular—found in fresh juice function as components of nerve cells, cellular membranes, and hormone-like substances called prostaglandins. They are also required for energy production. You can get more essential fatty acids by eating cold-water fish, flaxseed, walnuts, or other foods.

Vitamins. Fresh juice is loaded with vitamins. Along with minerals and enzymes, vitamins take part in chemical reactions. For example, vitamin C participates in the production of collagen, one of the main types of protein found in the body. Fresh juices are excellent sources of water-soluble vitamins such as C, many of the B vitamins, some fat-soluble vitamins such as vitamin E, and the carotenes, known as provitamin A (which are converted to vitamin A as needed by the body), and vitamin K.

Minerals. Fresh juice is loaded with minerals. There are about two dozen minerals that your body needs to function well. Minerals, along with vitamins, are components of enzymes. They make up part of bone, teeth, and blood tissue, and they help maintain normal cellular function. The major minerals include calcium, chloride, magnesium, phosphorus, potassium, sodium, and sulfur. Trace minerals are those needed in very small amounts, which include boron, chromium, cobalt, copper, fluoride, manganese, nickel, selenium, vanadium, and zinc. Minerals occur in inorganic forms in the soil, and plants incorporate them into their tissues. As a part of this process, the minerals are combined with organic molecules into easily absorbable forms, which makes plant food an excellent dietary source of minerals. Juicing is believed to provide even better mineral absorption than whole vegetables because the process of juicing liberates minerals into a highly absorbable, easily digestible form.

Enzymes. Fresh juices are chock-full of enzymes—those "living" molecules that work, with vitamins and minerals, to speed up reactions necessary for vital functions in the body. Without enzymes, we would not have life in our cells. Enzymes are prevalent in raw foods, but heat, such as cooking and pasteurization, destroys them. All juices that are bottled, even if kept in store refrigerators, have to be pasteurized. Heat temperatures for pasteurization are required to be far above the limit of what would preserve the enzymes and vitamins. When you eat and drink enzyme-rich foods, these little proteins help break down food in the digestive tract, thereby sparing the pancreas, small intestine, gallbladder, and stomach—the body's enzyme-producers—from overwork. This sparing action is known as the "law of adaptive secretion of digestive enzymes." This means that when a portion of the food you eat is digested by enzymes present in the food you ingest, the body will secrete less of its own enzymes, thus allowing your body's energy to be shifted from digestion to other functions such as repair and rejuvenation. In other words, fresh juices require very little energy expenditure to digest. And that is one reason why people who start consistently drinking fresh juice often report that they feel better and more energized right away.

Phytochemicals. Plants contain substances that protect them from disease, injury, and pollution. These substances are known as phytochemicals—*phyto* means plant and *chemical* in this context means nutrient. There are tens of thousands of phytochemicals in the foods we eat. For example, the average tomato may contain up to ten thousand different types of phytochemicals; the most famous being lycopene. Phytochemicals give plants their color, odor, and flavor. Unlike vitamins and enzymes, they are heat stable and can withstand cooking. Researchers have found that people who eat the most fruits and vegetables, which are the best sources of phytochemicals, have the lowest incidence of cancer and other diseases. Drinking vegetable juices gives you these vital substances in a concentrated form.

The Why and How of Juicing

Why juice? Why not just eat the fruits and vegetables?

Though I always tell people to eat their vegetables and fruit, there are at least three reasons why juicing is important and should also be included in the diet. First, we can juice far more produce than we would probably eat in a day. It takes a long time to chew raw veggies! Chewing is a very good thing, and I highly encourage it. However, we have only so much time for chewing up raw foods. One day I timed how long it would take for me to eat five medium-size carrots. (That's what I often juice along with cucumber, lemon, ginger root, beet, kale, and celery.) It took about fifty minutes to chew them up and swallow them. Not only do I not have that kind of time every day, but my jaw was also so tired afterward that I could hardly move it.

Second, we can juice parts of the plant we would not normally eat, such as stems, leaves, and seeds. I juice things I know I would rarely or never eat such as beet stems and leaves, celery leaves, the white pithy part of the lemon with the seeds, asparagus stems, broccoli stems, the base of cauliflower, kohlrabi leaves, radish leaves, and ribs of kale.

Third, juice is broken down so it spares digestion. It is estimated that it is at work in the system within twenty to thirty minutes. For ailments such as thyroid disorders, juice is therapy for this very reason. When the body has to work hard to break down veggies, it can spend a lot of energy on the digestive process. But juicing does the work for you. When you drink a glass of fresh juice, all those life-giving nutrients can go to work right away to heal and repair your body, giving it energy for its work of rejuvenation.

People often ask me if it takes a bushel basket full of produce to make a glass of juice. Actually, if you're using a good juicer, it takes a surprisingly small amount. For example, five to seven large carrots or one large cucumber yield about one eight-ounce glass of juice. The following amounts of produce each yield about four ounces of juice: one large apple, three to four large (thirteen-inch) ribs of celery, or one large orange. The key is to get a good juicer that yields a dry pulp. I've used juicers that ejected very wet pulp. When I ran the pulp through the juicer again, I got more juice, and the pulp was still wet.

GUIDELINES FOR JUICING

- Wash all produce before juicing. Fruit and vegetable washes are available at many grocery and health food stores. Or you can use hydrogen peroxide and then rinse. Cut away all moldy, bruised, or damaged areas of the produce.

- Always peel oranges, tangerines, tangelos, and grapefruit before juicing because the skins of these citrus fruit contain volatile oils that can cause digestive problems such as a stomachache. Lemon and lime peels can be juiced, if organic, but they do add a distinct flavor that you may not like. Peel them, but leave as much of the white pithy part on the citrus fruit as possible, since it contains the most vitamin C and bioflavonoids. Always peel mangoes and papayas, since their skins contain an irritant that is harmful when eaten in quantity. Peel all produce that is not labeled organic, even though the largest concentration of nutrients is found in and next to the skin. The peels and skins of sprayed fruits and vegetables contain the largest concentration of pesticides.

- Remove pits, stones, and hard seeds from fruits such as peaches, plums, apricots, cherries, and mangoes. Softer seeds from cucumbers, oranges, lemons, limes, watermelons, cantaloupes, grapes, papaya, and apples can be juiced without a problem.

- You can juice the stems and leaves of most produce such as beet stems and leaves, strawberry caps, celery leaves, and small grape stems; they offer nutrients too. Discard larger grape stems, as they can dull the juicer blade. Also remove carrot tops and rhubarb greens because they contain toxic substances. Cut off the ends of carrots since this is the part that molds first.

- Cut fruits and vegetables into sections or chunks that will fit your juicer's feed tube. You'll learn from experience what can be added whole or what size works best for your machine. If you have a large feed tube, you won't have to cut up a lot of produce.

- Drink and enjoy!

Some fruits and vegetables don't juice well. Most produce contains a lot of water, which is ideal for juicing. The vegetables and fruits that contain less water, such as bananas and avocados, will not juice well. They can be used in smoothies and cold soups by first juicing other produce, then pouring the juice into a blender, and adding the avocado, for example, to make a raw soup. Mangoes and papayas will juice but make a thicker juice.

Drink your juice as soon as you can after it's made. If you can't drink the juice right away, store it in an insulated container such as a thermos or another airtight, opaque container, and in the refrigerator. You can also freeze it.

Be aware that the longer juice sits before you drink it, the more nutrients are lost. If juice turns brown, it has oxidized and lost a large amount of its nutritional value; it is not good to drink it at this point as it may be spoiled. Melon and cabbage juice do not store well; drink them soon after they've been juiced.

Now that you've learned how to do it, it is time to dive in and make your first thyroid elixir!

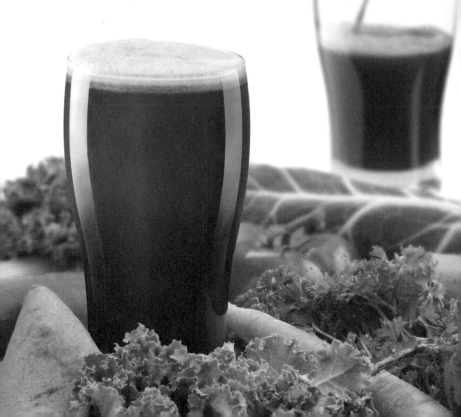

JUICE, SMOOTHIE, AND LIVING FOODS RECIPES TO HEAL YOUR THYROID

Juices

Adrenal Booster Cocktail

Hot peppers and parsley are rich in vitamin C; celery is a great source of natural sodium. Both are very beneficial for the adrenal glands.

1 handful of parsley
1 dark green lettuce leaf
4 carrots, scrubbed well, tops removed, ends trimmed
2 tomatoes
2 ribs of celery with leaves
Dash of hot sauce
Dash of Celtic sea salt

Cut produce to fit your juicer's feed tube. Wrap the parsley in the lettuce leaf and push through the juicer slowly. Juice all remaining ingredients, add hot sauce and sea salt, and stir. Pour into a glass and drink as soon as possible. Serves 2.

Alkaline Power

3 carrots, scrubbed well, tops removed, ends trimmed
2 ribs of celery with leaves
1 handful of spinach
1 cucumber, peeled if not organic
½ green apple

Cut produce to fit your juicer's feed tube. Juice all ingredients and stir. Pour into a glass and drink as soon as possible. Serves 1.

Arugula Cocktail

Pound for pound arugula is one of the most potent anticancer foods. Some of its phytochemicals, such as glucosinolate and sulforaphane, are responsible for stimulating enzymes that help the body cleanse away toxins and carcinogens. It also contains carotenes that can protect against sun damage, heart disease, and cancer. In addition, these nutrients improve communication between cells, something that may play a large role in healthy cellular function.

1 cucumber, peeled if not organic
1 handful of arugula
2 stalks celery
1-inch chunk ginger root
1 lemon, peeled if not organic

Cut cucumber in half. Juice one-half cucumber. Bunch up arugula and push through juicer with other half of the cucumber, followed by celery, ginger root, and lemon. Stir the juice and drink as soon as possible. Serves 1.

Asian Delight

1 chunk of jicama, approximately 2 inches by 4–5 inches, scrubbed well or peeled
2–3 carrots, scrubbed well, tops removed, ends trimmed

1 daikon radish, trimmed and scrubbed
1-inch chunk ginger root

Cut produce to fit your juicer's feed tube. Juice ingredients and stir. Pour into a glass and drink as soon as possible. Serves 1.

Beet Express

3 carrots, scrubbed well, tops removed, ends trimmed
2 kale leaves
1 small beet with green leaves
1-inch chunk ginger root
1 lemon, peeled if not organic
1 clove garlic

Cut produce to fit your juicer's feed tube. Juice all ingredients, stir, and drink as soon as possible. Serves 1.

Fitness Combo

1 handful of parsley
1 handful of spinach
2 lettuce leaves
3–4 carrots, scrubbed well, tops removed, ends trimmed
1 small beet with greens
1 rib of celery with leaves
¼ green pepper
2 cloves garlic
1-inch chunk ginger root

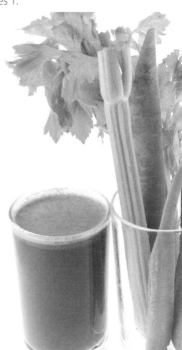

Wrap parsley and spinach in lettuce leaves. Cut all ingredients to fit your juicer's feed tube and push lettuce wraps through the juicer with remaining ingredients. Stir and serve as soon as possible. Serves 2.

Goin' Green

4 beet leaves
4 kohlrabi leaves
2 ribs of celery with leaves
1 cucumber, peeled if not organic
2–3 carrots, scrubbed well, tops removed, ends trimmed
1 pear
½ lemon

Place some green leaves in your juicer and alternate leaves with celery followed by cucumber, carrot, pear, and lemon. Stir the juice and drink as soon as possible. Serves 1–2.

Gourmet Live

1 small handful of parsley
1 cup loosely packed baby spinach leaves
3 dark green lettuce leaves
4 carrots, scrubbed well, green tops removed, ends trimmed
½ green pepper including seeds and inner membrane
2 green onions
1 garlic clove (no need to peel)
2 ribs of celery with leaves
½ small beet with leaves

Cut produce to fit your juicer's feed tube. Wrap parsley and spinach in lettuce leaves and push through the juicer followed by the remaining ingredients. Pour into glasses and drink as soon as possible. Serves 2.

Green Goddess

2 ribs of celery with leaves
1 cucumber, peeled if not organic
3 leaves dino kale
1 fennel stalk with fronds
6 sprigs parsley

Cut produce to fit your juicer's feed tube. Juice ingredients and stir. Pour into a glass and drink as soon as possible. Serves 1.

Green Recharger

1 cucumber, peeled if not organic
1 handful of sunflower sprouts
1 handful of buckwheat sprouts
1 small handful of clover sprouts
1 kale leaf
1 large handful of spinach
1 lime, peeled if not organic

Cut the cucumber to fit your juicer's feed tube. Juice half of the cucumber first. Bunch up the sprouts and wrap in the kale leaf. Turn off the machine and add them. Turn the machine back on and tap with the rest of the cucumber to gently push the sprouts and kale through followed by spinach. Then juice the remaining cucumber and lime. Stir ingredients, pour into a glass, and drink as soon as possible. Serves 1–2.

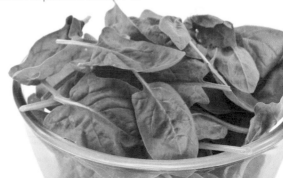

Green Supreme

2 ribs of celery with leaves
1 cucumber, peeled if not organic
1 chard leaf
1 handful of parsley
1 small handful of cilantro
1 green apple
1 lemon, peeled if not organic
1-inch chunk ginger root

Cut produce to fit your juicer's feed tube. Wrap parsley and cilantro in chard leaf. Start with celery and cucumber, push the chard-parsley-cilantro wrap through slowly and follow with remaining ingredients. Pour into a glass and drink as soon as possible. Serves 2.

Garlic Surprise

1 dark green lettuce leaf
1 handful of parsley
½ medium cucumber, peeled if not organic
1 garlic clove
3 carrots, scrubbed well, green tops removed, ends trimmed
2 ribs of celery with leaves

Wrap the parsley in the lettuce leaf. Juice the cucumber, the parsley-lettuce wrap, add the garlic and push through the juicer with the carrots, followed by the celery. Stir and pour into a glass and drink as soon as possible. Serves 1–2.

Lean Mean Green Juice

2 ribs of celery with leaves
1 cucumber, peeled if not organic
1 handful of spinach
1 handful of parsley
2 kale leaves
1-inch chunk ginger root
½ pear
½ green apple

Cut produce to fit your juicer's feed tube. Wrap parsley and spinach in kale leaves. Start with celery and cucumber, push the kale wraps through slowly and follow with remaining ingredients. Pour into a glass and drink as soon as possible. Serves 2.

Magnesium Special

4–5 beet tops
2 Swiss chard leaves
2 collard leaves
1 cucumber, peeled if not organic
½ green apple (omit if diabetic)
½ lemon, peeled if not organic

Cut produce to fit your juicer's feed tube. Juice ingredients and stir. Pour into a glass and drink as soon as possible. Serves 2.

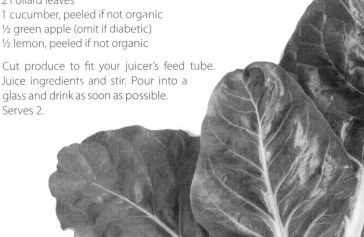

Misty Garden

3 carrots, scrubbed well, tops removed, ends trimmed
2–3 kale leaves
1 small handful of parsley
1 apple
1-inch chunk ginger root

Cut produce to fit your juicer's feed tube. Wrap parsley in a kale leaf. Start with carrots, push the kale wrap through slowly and follow with remaining ingredients. Pour into a glass and drink as soon as possible. Serves 1.

Moroccan Beet

1 beet, with leaves
1 cucumber, peeled if not organic
1 small bunch mint
1 lettuce leaf
1 lemon, peeled if not organic

Cut produce to fit your juicer's feed tube. Wrap mint in lettuce leaf. Start with beet and cucumber, push the lettuce-mint wrap through slowly and follow with remaining ingredients. Pour into a glass and drink as soon as possible. Serves 1.

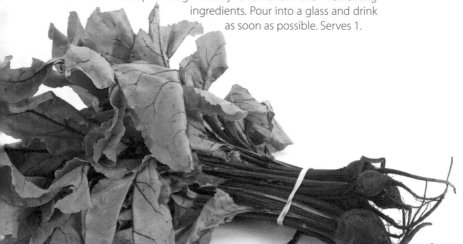

Mustard Surprise

Mustard greens provide what's known as "hot energy" in Chinese medicine. It promotes good circulation and relieves congestion.

3 carrots, scrubbed well, tops removed, ends trimmed
2 stalks celery
2–3 mustard leaves
1 cucumber, peeled if not organic
1 apple (green is lower in sugar)

Juice carrots and celery, roll mustard leaves and place in juicer. Push the greens through with the cucumber and apple. Stir the juice and drink as soon as possible. Serves 1–2.

Perky Parsley

3 carrots, scrubbed well, tops removed, ends trimmed
1 bunch parsley
2 dark green lettuce leaves
2 ribs of celery with leaves
1 cucumber, peeled if not organic
1 lemon, peeled if not organic

Cut produce to fit your juicer's feed tube. Wrap parsley in lettuce leaves and push through juicer slowly. Juice remaining ingredients and stir. Pour into a glass and drink as soon as possible. Serves 1–2.

Pineapple Kicker

¼ pineapple
6 kale leaves
2 ribs of celery with leaves
1-inch chunk ginger root

Cut produce to fit your juicer's feed tube. Juice ingredients and stir. Pour into a glass and drink as soon as possible. Serves 1.

Power Up

½ cucumber, peeled
1 small handful of parsley
1 green leaf lettuce leaf
3 carrots, scrubbed well, tops removed, ends trimmed
2 ribs of celery, with leaves as desired
½ beet, scrubbed well (may include stem and 1–2 leaves)
½ lemon, peeled if not organic

Cut produce to fit your juicer's feed tube. Start with cucumber. Wrap parsley in lettuce leaf and push through the machine slowly. Juice all remaining ingredients and stir. Pour into a glass and drink as soon as possible. Serves 1–2.

Red Sails in the Sunset

3 carrots, scrubbed well, tops removed, ends trimmed
½ red bell pepper with seeds and membrane
1 small beet with leaves
1 red Swiss chard leaf
1 lemon, peeled if not organic

Cut produce to fit your juicer's feed tube. Juice all ingredients and stir. Pour into a glass and drink as soon as possible. Serves 1.

Spicy Spinach-Grapefruit

1 cup fresh, loosely packed baby spinach
1 lettuce leaf
¼ medium jicama, peeled if not organic
½ red grapefruit, peeled
1-inch chunk ginger root

Cut produce to fit your juicer's feed tube. Wrap spinach in the lettuce leaf. Start with jicama, then push the lettuce wrap through slowly, and follow with remaining ingredients and stir. Juice ingredients and stir. Pour into a glass and drink as soon as possible. Serves 1.

Sprout-Cucumber Recharger

1 cucumber, peeled if not organic
1 large handful of spinach
2 kale leaves
1 handful of sunflower sprouts (optional)
1 handful of buckwheat sprouts (optional)
1 small handful of clover sprouts (optional)
1 lime, peeled if not organic

Cut the cucumber to fit your juicer's feed tube. Juice half of the cucumber first. Bunch up the sprouts and wrap in one kale leaf and the spinach in the other kale leaf. Turn off the machine and add them. Turn the machine back on and push through slowly with the rest of the cucumber, then juice the lime. Stir, pour into a glass, and drink as soon as possible. Serves 1–2.

Super Green

4 kale leaves
2 ribs of celery with leaves
1 cucumber, peeled if not organic
1 pear
1 lemon, peeled if not organic
1-inch chunk ginger root

Cut produce to fit your juicer's feed tube. Juice all ingredients and stir. Pour into a glass and drink as soon as possible. Serves 2.

Super Green II

1 small kohlrabi with leaves
1 kale leaf
1 kiwi fruit
1 rib of celery
1 apple (green has less sugar)
½ lemon, peeled

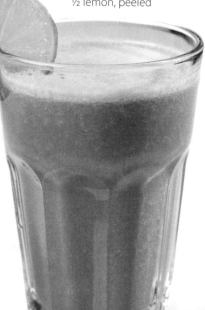

Cut produce to fit your juicer's feed tube. Roll the leaves and push through the juicer with the kiwi fruit and celery stalk. Add the apple and lemon and juice. Stir the juice and drink as soon as possible. Serves 1.

Super Green Sprout Drink

1 cucumber, peeled if not organic
1 rib of celery with leaves, as desired
1 small handful of sprouts such as broccoli or radish
1 large handful of sunflower sprouts
1 small handful of buckwheat sprouts
1 lemon, peeled if not organic

Cut produce to fit your juicer's feed tube. Juice all ingredients and stir. Pour into a glass and drink as soon as possible. Serves 1.

Super Sprout Drink

1 small handful of clover or radish sprouts
1 large handful of sunflower sprouts
1 small handful of buckwheat sprouts
2 kale leaves
1 organic cucumber, scrubbed well

Cut produce to fit your juicer's feed tube. Wrap sprouts in kale leaves and push through juicer slowly with the cucumber. Pour into a glass and drink as soon as possible. Serves 1.

Sweet Green Sombrero

1 red or yellow apple
3 carrots, scrubbed well, tops removed, ends trimmed
2 ribs of celery with leaves
2 kale leaves
1 cucumber, peeled if not organic
1 lemon, peeled
¼ jalapeño pepper, seeds removed unless you like it really hot

Cut produce to fit your juicer's feed tube. Start with apple and then juice all ingredients and stir. Pour into a glass and drink as soon as possible. Serves 2.

Sweet Serenity

1 handful of spinach
1 romaine leaf
1 apple
2 ribs of celery with leaves
1 cucumber, peeled if not organic
1 lime, peeled if not organic

Cut produce to fit your juicer's feed tube. Wrap spinach in the romaine leaf. Start with apple, then push the lettuce wrap through slowly, and follow with remaining ingredients and stir. Pour into a glass and drink as soon as possible. Serves 1.

The Morning Energizer

3–4 carrots, scrubbed well, tops removed, ends trimmed
1 cucumber, peeled if not organic
1 small beet, scrubbed well, with stems and leaves
1 lemon, peeled
1-inch chunk ginger root, peeled
½ green apple

Cut the produce to fit your juicer's feed tube. Juice all ingredients and stir. Pour into a glass and drink as soon as possible. Serves 1–2.

Thyroid Tonic I

Radishes are a traditional tonic for the thyroid. In the old Soviet Union black and red radishes were accepted and recommended by some doctors as a medical treatment for hypothyroidism. Radishes contain a sulphur component called raphanin that keeps the production of thyroxine and calcitonin (a peptide hormone) in normal balance.

5 carrots, scrubbed well, green tops removed, ends trimmed
½ medium lemon, peeled
5–6 radishes, with green tops

Cut produce to fit your juicer's feed tube. Juice ingredients and stir. Pour into a glass and drink as soon as possible. Serves 1.

Thyroid Tonic II

5–6 radishes, with green tops
1 carrot, scrubbed well, green top removed, ends trimmed
1 tomato
1 rib of celery or equivalent size chunk of zucchini
Pinch of kelp

Cut produce to fit your juicer's feed tube. Juice ingredients and stir. Pour into a glass and drink as soon as possible. Serves 1.

Twisted Ginger

4 carrots, scrubbed well, green tops removed, ends trimmed
1 handful of parsley
1 lemon, peeled
1 apple
2-inch chunk fresh ginger root, peeled

Cut produce to fit your juicer's feed tube. Juice ingredients and stir. Pour into a glass and drink as soon as possible. Serves 1–2.

Totally Green

    5 green leaf lettuce leaves
    1 handful of parsley
    1 handful of spinach
    2 ribs of celery with leaves
    2 green apples (for a little sweet taste)

Cut produce to fit your juicer's feed tube. Wrap the parsley and spinach in the lettuce leaves and push through the juicer slowly with the celery and apple. Stir the juice and drink as soon as possible. Serves 1.

Wild Green Energy Cocktail

Wild greens reduce the desire for starchy foods, thus making them an excellent weight-loss helper.

    1 cucumber, peeled if not organic
    1 rib of celery
    1 handful of wild greens such as dandelion, nettles, plantain,
        lamb's quarters, or sorrel
    1 apple (green is lower in sugar)
    1 lemon, peeled if not organic

Cut all ingredients to fit your juicer's feed tube. Juice all ingredients and stir. Pour into a glass and drink as soon as possible. Serves 1.

Smoothies

Avocado Cream

½ cup almond milk
1 avocado, peeled and seeded
1 handful of spinach
2 Tbsp. fresh lemon juice
2–3 drops stevia
1 tsp. pure vanilla extract
1 tsp. freshly grated organic lemon peel
6 ice cubes

Combine all ingredients in a blender and process well until smooth and creamy. Serve chilled. Serves 1.

Caribbean Morning

1 cup coconut milk
½ cup fresh orange juice
1 Tbsp. coconut oil
1½ cups fresh or frozen papaya chunks
1 cup fresh or frozen pineapple chunks
½ cup chopped kale
2 Tbsp. unsweetened shredded coconut
6 ice cubes (optional; not needed if using fresh fruit)

Pour the coconut milk, orange juice, and coconut oil in a blender and blend. Then add the papaya, pineapple, kale, shredded coconut and ice cubes; blend until smooth. Serves 2.

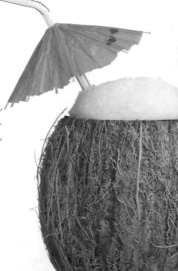

Cherie's Green Morning Blend

½ English cucumber, peeled and cut into chunks
1 avocado, peeled, seeded, and cut in quarters
1 cup loosely packed baby spinach
Juice of 1 lime
1 Tbsp. green powder of choice (optional)
2–3 Tbsp. ground almonds (optional)

Combine all ingredients except almonds in a blender and blend well. Sprinkle ground almonds on top, as desired. Serves 1.

Cranberry-Pear Fat Buster

2 pears, Bartlett or Asian
1 cucumber, peeled if not organic
½ cup loosely packed baby spinach
¼ lemon, peeled if not organic
2 Tbsp. cranberries, fresh or frozen
½–1-inch chunk ginger root
6 ice cubes (optional)

Chop up pears and cucumber and blend until smooth. Add spinach, lemon, cranberries, ginger, and ice as desired, and blend until creamy. Serves 1.

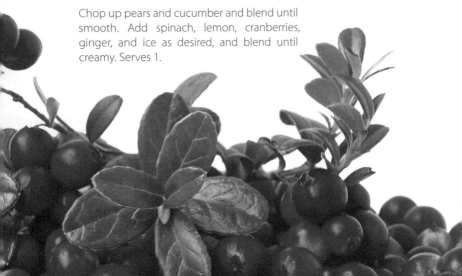

Dandelion Morning

½ bunch dandelion greens
2 ribs of celery with leaves
1-inch chunk fresh ginger root
1 peach, seed removed
1 cup berries, fresh or frozen

Combine all ingredients in a blender and process until smooth and creamy. Serves 2.

Fat Burner

Ginger root helps raise metabolism, which helps you burn more calories.

1 cup carrot juice
1 apple, cut into chunks
1 banana, peeled and cut into chunks
1 cup (packed) baby spinach
1-inch chunk ginger root
6 ice cubes

Place all ingredients in a blender and process until smooth. Pour into glasses and serve chilled. Serves 2.

Green Berry Delight

1 cucumber, peeled if not organic
½ apple
1 cup berries (blueberries, raspberries, or blackberries), fresh or
    thawed if frozen
3–4 dark green leaves (collards, Swiss chard, or kale)
1-inch chunk ginger root
Juice of ½ lemon
1 avocado, peeled, seeded, and cut into chunks

Cut the cucumber and apple in chunks. Place the cucumber,
apple, and berries in a blender and process until smooth. Chop
the greens and ginger and add to the blender along with the
lemon juice and avocado. Process until well blended. Serves 2.

Green Mint Dream

1 cup plain yogurt
2 cups cucumber, peeled and diced
1 handful of spinach
2 Tbsp. scallions, chopped
½ tsp. Celtic sea salt
¼ cup chopped mint leaves
1 garlic clove, peeled and minced

Combine all ingredients in a
blender and process on high
speed until smooth. Pour into
bowls and serve immediately.
Serves 2.

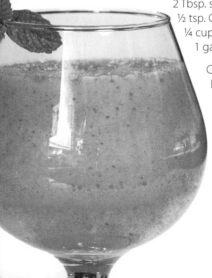

Guava-Pineapple Flip

1 cup coconut milk
1 cup guava nectar
1 cup fresh or frozen pineapple chunks
1 frozen banana, cut into chunks
½ cup loosely packed baby spinach
1 tsp. pure vanilla extract
6 ice cubes (optional: not needed if using frozen fruit)

Combine all ingredients in a blender and process until smooth and creamy. Pour into glasses and serve immediately. Serves 2.

Green Piña Colada

½ cup coconut milk
1 cup fresh pineapple, peeled and diced
¼ cup lightly packed grated coconut
1 handful of spinach
1 tsp. pure vanilla extract
4–5 drops liquid stevia
1 banana, peeled and cut into chunks
6 ice cubes

Combine all ingredients in a blender and process on high speed until smooth. Pour into glasses and serve immediately. Serves 2.

Healthy Green Smoothie

1 cucumber, peeled if not organic
2 stalks celery
1 handful of kale, parsley, or spinach
1 green apple
½ lemon, peeled if not organic
6 ice cubes

Chop the cucumber, celery, greens, and apple. Place in blender with lemon and ice; process until creamy. Serves 2.

Razzmatazz

1 cup fresh orange juice
1 banana, peeled and cut into chunks
1 cup loosely packed baby spinach
½ cup raspberries, fresh or frozen
½ cup blueberries, fresh or frozen
½ cup blackberries, fresh or frozen
3 ice cubes, if using frozen fruit; 6 ice cubes if using fresh fruit

Place all ingredients in a blender and blend until smooth. Pour into glasses and serve chilled. Serves 2.

Sail Away

1 papaya, peeled and cut into chunks
(about 1½ cups); you may use a few seeds
1 cup packed baby spinach
¾ cup coconut milk
¼ cup grated unsweetened coconut, lightly packed
1½ tsp. freshly grated lime peel, organic
1 tsp. pure vanilla extract

Combine all ingredients in a blender and process until smooth and creamy. Serve immediately. Serves 1.

Southwestern Green Smoothie

1¼ cups fresh carrot juice (5–7 medium, or approx. 1 lb., yield
about 1 cup)
1 handful of spinach
1 avocado, peeled, seeded, and cut into chunks
½ tsp. ground cumin

Juice carrots and pour the juice in a blender. Add the spinach,
avocado, and cumin and blend until smooth. Serve chilled.
Serves 1–2.

Spice Girl

1 cup fresh green apple juice (about two apples)
1 banana, peeled and cut into chunks
1-inch chunk ginger root (juice with the apples or grate)
4 oz. soft silken organic tofu
½ cup packed baby spinach
½ tsp. cinnamon
⅛ tsp. ground black pepper
⅛ tsp. ground cumin
⅛ tsp. ground cardamom

Combine all ingredients in a blender and process until smooth
and creamy. Pour into glasses and serve chilled. Serves 2.

Strawberry Coconut Cream

½ cup almond milk
5 oz. soft silken organic tofu
⅓ cup grated coconut, lightly packed
8–10 strawberries, fresh or frozen
½ cup loosely packed baby spinach
1 tsp. pure vanilla extract
6 ice cubes

Place all ingredients in a blender and process until creamy and smooth. Serve chilled. Serves 1.

Strawberry Shangri-La

½ cup fresh orange juice
1 lb. strawberries with caps (about 1 quart)
1 ripe banana, cut into chunks
1 handful of spinach
½ cup silken organic tofu
6–8 ice cubes

Juice an orange and pour the juice in a blender. Add the remaining ingredients and blend until smooth. Serve cold. Serves 2.

Super Green Smoothie

1¼ cups fresh cucumber juice (about 1 large or 2 medium
    cucumbers, peeled if not organic)
2 ribs of celery with leaves, juiced
1 kale leaf, chopped
1 avocado, peeled, seeded, and cut into chunks
1 garlic clove, peeled
4 oz. soft silken organic tofu
½ cup flat-leaf parsley, coarsely chopped
2 tsp. sweet onion, minced
1 tsp. dried dill weed

Pour the cucumber and celery juices into a blender and add
the kale, avocado, garlic, tofu, parsley, onion, and dill. Blend on
high speed until smooth and creamy; serve immediately, as it
does not taste good if it sits. Serves 2.

Tropical Frosty

1 cup fresh pineapple, chopped
1 orange, torn in segments
1 frozen banana, cut into chunks
1 cup fresh strawberries with caps
1 cup packed baby spinach
Juice of 1 lemon
Juice of 1 orange
6–8 ice cubes
Ground almonds or chia seeds (optional as a garnish)

Place all ingredients in a blender and process until smooth
and creamy. Pour into glasses, sprinkle ground almonds or chia
seeds on top, and serve chilled. Serves 2.

Tropical Treat

1 papaya, peeled, seeds removed, cut into chunks (about 1½ cups), frozen
¾ cup coconut water
1½ tsp. freshly grated orange peel, organic
1 tsp. pure vanilla extract
1 cup spinach

Place the papaya chunks in a freezer bag and freeze them until solid. Pour the milk into a blender and add the papaya, orange peel, vanilla, and spinach. Blend on high speed until smooth and serve immediately. Serves 2.

Weight-Loss Partner

1 cup coconut milk
1 cup berries of choice
½ cup packed baby spinach
1–2 Tbsp. protein powder of choice
1 Tbsp. virgin organic coconut oil
1 Tbsp. ground flaxseeds
1 tsp. pure vanilla extract
¼ tsp. almond extract
2–3 drops stevia
6–8 ice cubes

Combine all ingredients but ice in a blender and process until creamy and smooth. Add ice after the coconut oil is blended so that it won't clump. You may use more or less ice, depending on how cold you like your smoothie. Serves 1–2.

Living Foods Recipes

Breakfast

Apple Muesli

Oats are a good source of B vitamins, vitamin F, manganese, zinc, selenium, nickel, molybdenum, and vanadium. Oats contain gluten (substitute buckwheat groats, if gluten sensitive) and phytates, a binding agent that can cause some mineral loss if consumed frequently.

Soaking grains overnight, as recommended here, breaks down some of the phytic acid in the bran.

½ cup raisins
¼ cup rolled oats
2 Tbsp. sunflower seeds
2 Tbsp. flaxseeds
2 Tbsp. bee pollen
½ tsp. ascorbic acid (vitamin C powder)
½ cup milk of choice
½ cup chopped apple
½ tsp. cinnamon extract or ground cinnamon

Place raisins, oats, sunflower seeds, flaxseeds, bee pollen, and ascorbic acid in a bowl and cover with milk. Cover the bowl and let soak overnight in the refrigerator. Add chopped apple and cinnamon before serving. Makes about 1½ cups.

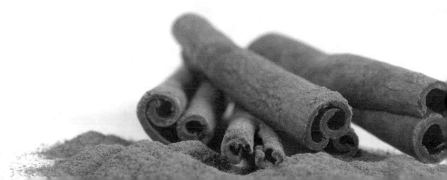

Lemon Muesli

Flaxseeds are rich in omega-3 fatty acids and are one of the richest sources of lignans. To release these heart-healthy nutrients from the hard coating of the flaxseed, it must be ground in a blender or nut grinder. Otherwise the flaxseed will pass right through your body without much benefit.

¼ cup rolled oats
¼ cup raisins
2 Tbsp. almonds
2 Tbsp. flaxseeds
½ tsp. ascorbic acid (vitamin C powder)
½ cup milk of choice
1 Tbsp. fresh lemon juice
1 tsp. freshly grated lemon peel, preferably organic

Place the oats, raisins, almonds, flaxseeds, and vitamin C in a bowl; pour the milk over them. Cover the bowl and refrigerate overnight. Add the lemon juice and zest before serving and stir. Makes about 1 cup.

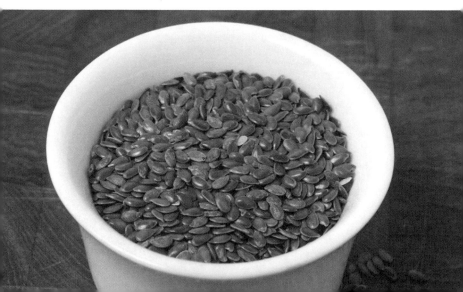

Sprouted Buckwheat Groats

Put 1 cup (or as much as you want) of raw buckwheat groat seeds into a bowl or your sprouter. Add 2–3 times as much cool, purified water. Swish seeds around to ensure even water contact for all. Allow seeds to soak for 6–8 hours. Drain off the soak water. Rinse thoroughly with cool water. Groats create very starchy water; it's very thick! They won't sprout well unless rinsed well, so rinse until the water runs clear. Drain thoroughly. You can add to your sprouter at this time or simply put the sprouts in a colander and cover with a tea towel. Set out of direct sunlight at room temperature (70 degrees is optimal). Rinse and drain again in 4–8 hours. Yields approximately 1½ cups of sprouts.

For your morning cereal, sprouted buckwheat is great served with rice, oat, or almond milk and a sprinkle of ground almonds and cinnamon. You can also dehydrate sprouted groats for a crunchy cereal.

Salads

Apple Fennel Salad With Lemon Zest

2 cups fennel, sliced julienne thin
2 cups apple, sliced julienne thin
2 Tbsp. fresh lemon juice
2 Tbsp. lemon zest
2 Tbsp. extra-virgin olive oil
2 Tbsp. fresh, minced thyme
1 sliver of jalapeño, minced
1 tsp. Celtic sea salt

Place the fennel and apple slices in a bowl; set aside. In a small bowl, whisk together lemon juice, zest, olive oil, thyme, jalapeño, and salt. Pour dressing over fennel-apple mixture and toss. Serves 4.

Winter Salad

1 large grapefruit
2 small fresh fennel bulbs, trimmed, halved vertically, sliced paper-thin (save discarded parts for juicing)
1 cup fresh parsley, chopped
Lemon-Ginger Dressing

Peel grapefruit and cut off white part. Separate segments and slice into pieces. Combine grapefruit, fennel, and parsley. Add dressing to taste and toss. Serves 2.

Lemon-Ginger Dressing

2 lemons, juiced
2-inch chunk ginger root, grated
½ cup extra-virgin olive oil
2 cloves garlic, peeled and crushed
3 Tbsp. miso
2 Tbsp. shoyu
2–3 Tbsp. raw honey or pure maple syrup

Mix all ingredients in blender. If needed, add water to thin. Makes 1 cup.

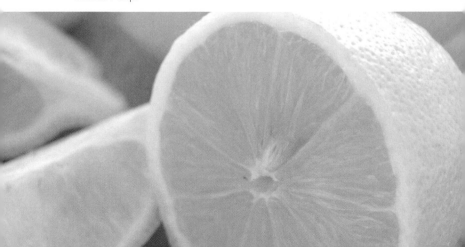

Sprouted Quinoa Salad

Quinoa is a seed, not a grain, but it can substitute for any grain. It is high in protein, complete with all eight essential amino acids, and it's gluten free.

2 cups sprouted quinoa
2 avocados, diced
2 tomatoes, diced
1 clove garlic, minced
½ cup chopped cilantro (optional)
3 Tbsp. nutritional yeast
1 tsp. cumin
½ tsp. Celtic sea salt
Juice of 1 lime

Soak quinoa overnight and then sprout for two days. Put quinoa in a bowl with remaining ingredients. Toss and serve on a bed of greens or in raw burritos. Serves 4.

Ginger-Beet Salad

4 cups grated beets
1 Tbsp. grated ginger root
¼ cup extra-virgin olive oil
¼ cup fresh lemon juice

Finely grate beets in food processor or with grater. In small bowl, combine beets, ginger, olive oil, and lemon juice. Toss and let the flavors blend for a few minutes before serving. Serves 4.

Main Courses

Raw Zucchini Noodles With Marinara Sauce

6 to 8 firm zucchini and/or yellow crookneck squash
1 cup Marinara Sauce
Fresh basil, chopped, to taste (optional)
Avocado slices (optional)

Use a vegetable spiral slicer or spirooli to make thin, long noodles out of zucchini. If possible, make zucchini noodles about six hours before serving, and let noodles sit in a bowl, uncovered, at room temperature, which can improve their texture.

Pour Marinara Sauce over the noodles, give the noodles and sauce a good toss, and serve. Top with chopped fresh basil and/or slices of avocado. Serves 3 to 4.

You can also use Raw Pesto Sauce. Or you can make my favorite—a simple pasta dish of zucchini noodles tossed with several tablespoons of extra-virgin olive oil, 2–3 cloves of pressed garlic, ¼ cup halved sun-dried olives, and ¼ cup chopped fresh basil. Sprinkle with salt, to taste, and serve.

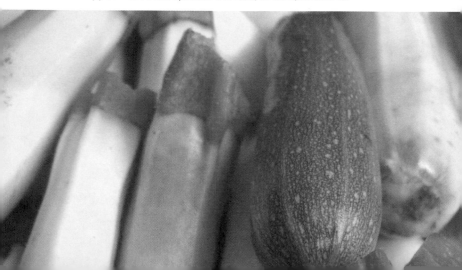

Marinara Sauce

1 cup sun-dried tomatoes
1½ cups blended tomatoes
2 Tbsp. chopped onion
2 garlic cloves, peeled
2 Tbsp. extra-virgin olive oil
½ cup fresh lemon juice
Celtic sea salt, to taste

Combine all the ingredients in a blender and process until desired consistency is reached. Makes about 3 cups.

Raw Pesto Sauce

½–¾ cup organic raw pine nuts
¼ cup fresh organic basil, de-stemmed
2 Tbsp. extra-virgin olive oil
1–2 Tbsp. fresh lemon juice
1–2 garlic cloves
1 tsp. Celtic sea salt
¼ cup purified water, reserved

Add all the ingredients to a food processor or blender. Pulse the mixture in food processor or blender, adding 1 tablespoon of water at a time to help facilitate blending and in order to reach the desired consistency for the sauce. Makes about 1¼ cups.

Nan's Sunflower Pate

Sunflower seeds are an excellent source of vitamin E, the body's primary fat-soluble antioxidant. Vitamin E has significant anti-inflammatory effects that result in the reduction of symptoms in asthma, osteoarthritis, and rheumatoid arthritis, conditions where free radicals and inflammation play a big role.

3 cups sunflower seeds, soaked 8–12 hours; rinse and sprout
    about 4 hours
1 cup fresh lemon juice
½ cup scallions, chopped
¼–½ cup raw tahini
¼ cup liquid aminos or shoyu
2–4 slices red onion, cut into chunks
4–6 Tbsp. parsley, chopped
2–3 medium cloves garlic
½ tsp. cayenne pepper
1–2 Tbsp. ginger, chopped
1 tsp. ground cumin

Blend all ingredients in food processor until all the ingredients are smooth and creamy. This mixture should be on the thick side rather than thin. Add a bit of water as needed. Makes 7–8 cups.

Almond Falafel

3 cups almonds, soaked
1½ cups sunflower seeds, soaked
Juice of 2 lemons
4 cloves garlic, finely chopped
½ cup raw tahini
1½ Tbsp. curry
3 cups of greens such as parsley, cilantro, or kale, finely chopped
    (use food processor or finely mince)

Soak nuts and seeds for several hours. Put drained, soaked almonds in food processor and chop fine. Set aside in a medium bowl. Process the soaked sunflower seeds and put in the bowl, adding lemon juice. Add garlic, tahini, curry, and greens. Mix everything together and massage with hands. Shape into small patties and serve fresh, or dehydrate at 105 degrees for 4–5 hours. Serve with the Sunflower Dill Sauce. Makes 6 servings.

Sunflower Dill Sauce

2 cups raw sunflower seeds, soaked for 8–12
    hours
⅔ cup lemon juice or 1 cucumber, peeled
⅓ cup extra-virgin olive oil
2 Tbsp. minced garlic
1 tsp. Celtic sea salt
6 Tbsp. fresh, chopped dill or 2 Tbsp. dried dill

In a high-speed blender, blend sunflower seeds, lemon juice or cucumber, olive oil, garlic, and salt until smooth. Pulse in the dill. More cucumber may be added for desired consistency if needed. Makes about 3–3¼ cups.

Carrot Sauce With Asparagus and Fresh Peas Over Rice

1 cup brown rice or quinoa
1½ cups carrot juice (about 8–11 carrots)
½ cup raw cashews
2 Tbsp. white or yellow miso
1 pound fresh asparagus
½ cup fresh or frozen peas
2 scallions, chopped
¼ cup marinated sun-dried tomato halves, thinly sliced
2 cloves garlic, pressed
3 Tbsp. fresh basil, finely chopped

Cook brown rice or quinoa according to directions.

While rice or quinoa is cooking, combine the carrot juice, cashews, and miso in a blender or food processor, blending on high until the cashews are no longer gritty and the mixture is smooth and creamy. Snap off the tops of the asparagus. Cut the tender upper portion into 1-inch pieces.

In a medium-size skillet, combine the carrot juice mixture and asparagus. Bring to a boil and then reduce the heat to simmer, stirring occasionally for 2–3 minutes. Add the peas and simmer until the asparagus is just tender, about 2 minutes. Add the scallions, sun-dried tomatoes, and garlic, mixing well; simmer for 1–2 minutes. Remove the sauce from the heat.

Divide the rice or quinoa in 4 portions. Top each portion with about ¼ of the sauce and sprinkle chopped basil on top of each portion. Serves 4.

Nicole's Stuffed Acorn Squash

1 acorn squash
½ cup grass-fed ground turkey
¼ cup quinoa
1–2 garlic cloves, pressed
1 tsp. dried basil
½–1 tsp. Celtic sea salt
½ tsp. cumin
½ tsp. paprika
Red bell pepper strips

Bake the acorn squash at 400 degrees for 20 minutes. Remove from oven; cut squash in half and scoop out seeds. Return to oven and bake for 25 minutes, or until tender. Adding a little water to the baking pan will speed the baking process.

While the squash is baking, cook the ground turkey and quinoa in separate pans. When cooked, scoop the turkey and quinoa into a bowl and add the basil, salt, cumin, and paprika. Stir until well combined. Scoop half the mixture into each half of the acorn squash. Top with several red bell pepper strips.

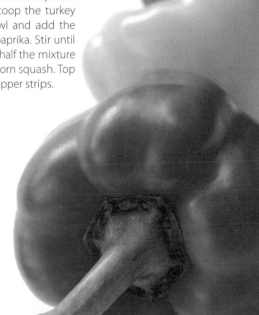

Healthy Desserts

Lemon Torte

1 cup cashews, soaked for 8 hours
2 lemons, zested
Juice of 2 lemons
2 Tbsp. pure maple syrup
1 orange, juiced
1 Tbsp. psyllium powder
Shortbread Crust (this page)

Blend all ingredients, except psyllium, in a blender until the mixture is the consistency of whipped cream. Fold in psyllium. Pour into Shortbread Crust, cover with Saran Wrap, and freeze for at least 1 hour. Take out of freezer and refrigerate 30 minutes before serving. Serves 4.

Shortbread Crust

2½ cups shredded coconut
½ cup cashews, soaked 1 hour
2 Tbsp. honey

Put coconut in blender and start on low speed, then high. As well forms, slowly add cashews to crumbly stage. Then add honey. Use spatula if needed to blend. Blend until mixture heats a little bit. Press crust in bottom and sides of 1 large or 4 small tart pans. Makes 4 small tarts or 1 large tart to use with your choice of fillings.

Summer Peach Parfait

7 peaches, peeled and thinly sliced
2 cups raw almonds, soaked in 3 cups purified water for 6–12 hours
4 Tbsp. raw almond butter
¼ cup honey or pure maple syrup
½ cup fresh orange juice
2 Tbsp. pure vanilla extract
2 tsp. cinnamon
4 tsp. nutmeg
Pinch Celtic sea salt
2 pints blueberries (optional)

Blend 1 peeled peach and remaining ingredients, except blueberries. Add more orange juice as needed to aid in blending until a custard consistency is reached. In parfait glasses, layer peaches, custard, peaches, custard; top with blueberries (if using). Serves 8.

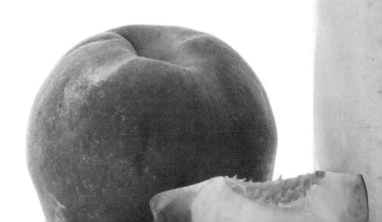

NOTES

Chapter 2
The Little Gland With Big Influence

1. Bodil-Cecilie Sondergaard et al., "The Effect of Oral Calcitonin on Cartilage Turnover and Surface Erosion in an Ovariectomized Rat Model," *Arthritis and Rheumatism* 56, no. 8 (August 2007): 2647–2678.

2. Na Li et al., "Dibutyl Phthalate Contributes to Thyroid Receptor Antagonistic Activity in Drinking Water Processes," *Environmental Science and Technology* 44, no. 17 (September 1, 2010): 6863–6868.

3. Kellyn S. Betts, "Thyroid Insult: Flame Retardants Linked to Alterations in Pregnant Women's TSH Levels," *Environmental Health Perspectives* 118, no. 10 (October 2010): 445.

4. Rachel A. Heimeier et al., "The Xenoestrogen Bisphenol A Inhibits Postembryonic Vertebrate Development by Antagonizing Gene Regulation by Thyroid Hormone," *Endocrinology* 150, no. 6 (June 2009): 2964–2943.

5. Lyn Patrick, "Thyroid Disruption: Mechanisms and Clinical Implications in Human Health," *Alternative Medicine Review* 14, no. 4 (December 2009): 326–346.

6. University of Exeter, "Stain Repellent Chemical Linked to Thyroid Disease in Adults," January 21, 2010, http://medicine.exeter.ac.uk/news/2010/title_53134_en.html (accessed February 18, 2015).

7. Environmental Working Group, "44 Million Women at Risk of Thyroid Deficiency From Rocket Fuel Chemical," news release, October 4, 2006, http://www.ewg.org/news/news-releases/2006/10/04/44-million-women-risk-thyroid-deficiency-rocket-fuel-chemical (accessed February 18, 2015).

8. Craig Steinmaus, Mark D. Miller, and Robert Howd, "Impact of Smoking and Thiocyanate on Perchlorate and Thyroid Hormone Associations in the 2001–2002 National Health and Nutrition Examination Survey," *Environmental Health Perspectives* 115, no. 9 (September 2007): 1333–1338.

9. L. Kotze et al., "Thyroid Disorders in Brazilian Patients With Celiac Disease," *Journal of Clinical Gastroenterology* 40, no. 1 (January 2006): 33–36.

10. Andrea McCreery, "How to Protect Yourself From Radiation Exposure," Life-Sources.com, March 17, 2011, http://www.life -sources.com/news/70/How-to-Protect-Yourself-from-Radiation -Exposure.html (accessed February 18, 2015).

11. Ahmet Koyua et al., "Effects of 900 MHz Electromagnetic Field on TSH and Thyroid Hormones in Rats," *Toxicology Letters* 157, nos. 3, 4 (July 2005): 257–262.

Chapter 3
Getting Back to Better Than Normal

1. Joseph Mercola, "McDonald's and Biophoton Deficiency," Mercola .com, August 21, 2002, http://articles.mercola.com/sites/articles/ archive/2002/08/21/biophoton.aspx (accessed February 18, 2015).

2. John Switzer, "Bio-Photon Nutrition and Wild Green Energy Cocktails for Optimal Health (English)," May 21, 2009, http://tinyurl .com/lkxqve4 (accessed February 18, 2015).

3. Tan Vinh, "Power Meals: Seahawks Chef Plays Key Role in Team's Success," *Seattle Times*, January 9, 2014, http://www.seattle times.com/seattle-news/power-meals-seahawks-chef-plays -key-role-in-teamrsquos-success/ (accessed February 24, 2015).

Chapter 4
What You Don't Know May Be Killing Your Thyroid

1. Ryan Robbins, "Are Nonstick Pans Linked to Thyroid Disease?", Bastyr University Health Tips, January 26, 2011, http://bastyr.edu/ news/news.asp?NewsID=2272 (accessed March 10, 2011).

2. *Environmental Health Perspectives*, "Stain Repellent Chemical Linked to Thyroid Disease in U.S. Adults."

3. Robbins, "Are Nonstick Pans Linked to Thyroid Disease?"

4. R. L. Divi, H. C. Chang, and D. R. Doerge, "Anti-Thyroid Isoflavones From Soybean: Isolation, Characterization, and Mechanisms of Action," *Biochemical Pharmacology* 54, no. 10 (November 15, 1997): 1087–1096.

5. Mary Shomon, "Do Soy Products Negatively Affect Your Thyroid?", Thyroid –Info.com, http://www.thyroid-inf0.com/articles/soy dangers.htm (accessed December 4, 2014).

6. P. Fort et al., "Breast and Soy-Formula Feeding in Early Infancy and the Prevalence of Autoimmune Thyroid Disease in Children," *Journal of the American College of Nutrition* 9, no. 2 (April 1990): 164–167.

7. Kotze, "Thyroid Disorders in Brazilian Patients With Celiac Disease."

8. Chris Kessler, "The Gluten-Thyroid Connection," http://chriskresser.com/the-gluten-thyroid-connection (accessed February 20, 2015).

9. Ibid.

10. Ibid.

11. S. Pavelka, "Metabolism of Bromide and Its Interference With the Metabolism of Iodine," *Physiological Research* 53, Suppl. 1 (2004): S80–S90.

12. Ibid.

13. C. Pelletier, P. Imbeault, and A. Tremblay, "Energy Balance and Pollution by Organochlorines and Polychlorinated Biphenyls," *Obesity Reviews* 4, no. 1 (February 2003): 17–24.

14. TruthAboutSplenda.com, "Frequently Asked Questions," http://www.truthaboutsplenda.com/resources/faqs.html (accessed February 20, 2015).

15. Deanna Dean, "An Underactive Thyroid May Be Cause of Your High Cholesterol," Naturalnews.com, May 19, 2010, http://www.naturalnews.com/028816_thyroid_high_cholesterol.html (accessed February 20, 2015).

Chapter 5

Nourish Your Thyroid With Living Foods

1. Sciencedaily.com, "Brain Chemical Boosts Body Heat, Aids in Calorie Burn, UT Southwestern Research Suggests," July 7, 2010, www.sciencedaily.com/releases/2010/07/100706123015.htm (accessed February 24, 2015).

2. ScienceDaily.com, "Peppers May Increase Energy Expenditure in People Trying to Lose Weight," April 28, 2010, http://www.sciencedaily.com/releases/2010/04/100427190934.htm (accessed February 24, 2015).

3. Environmental Working Group, "EWG's 2013 Shopper's Guide to Pesticides in Produce," http://www.ewg.org/foodnews/summary.php (accessed February 18, 2015).

4. Ibid.

FOR MORE INFORMATION

Sign up for the Juice Lady's free Juice Newsletter at www .juiceladycherie.com.

Cherie's website: www.juiceladycherie.com (information on juicing and weight loss)

The Juice Lady's health and wellness juice retreats

I invite you to join us for a week that can change your life! Our retreats offer gourmet organic raw foods with a three-day juice fast midweek. We offer interesting, informative classes in a beautiful, peaceful setting where you can experience healing and restoration of body and soul. For more information, a brochure, and dates for the retreats, call 866-843-8935.

Schedule a nutrition consultation with the Juice Lady: Call 866-8GETWEL (866-843-8935).

Juicers

Find out the best juicers recommended by Cherie Calbom. Call 866-8GETWEL (866-843-8935) or visit http://www.juice ladycherie.com/Juice/store/.

Dehydrators

Find out the best dehydrators recommended by Cherie Calbom. Call 866-8GETWEL (866-843-8935) or visit http:// www.juiceladycherie.com/Juice/store/.